Palgrave Texts in Counselling and Psychotherapy

Series Editors
Arlene Vetere, Family Therapy and Systemic Practice, VID
Specialized University, Oslo, Norway
Rudi Dallos, Clinical Psychology, Plymouth University,
Plymouth, UK

This series introduces readers to the theory and practice of counselling and psychotherapy across a wide range of topical issues. Ideal for both trainees and practitioners, the books will appeal to anyone wishing to use counselling and psychotherapeutic skills and will be particularly relevant to workers in health, education, social work and related settings. The books in this series emphasise an integrative orientation weaving together a variety of models including, psychodynamic, attachment, trauma, narrative and systemic ideas. The books are written in an accessible and readable style with a focus on practice. Each text offers theoretical background and guidance for practice, with creative use of clinical examples.

Arlene Vetere, Professor of Family Therapy and Systemic Practice at VID Specialized University, Oslo, Norway.

Rudi Dallos, Emeritus Professor, Dept. of Clinical Psychology, University of Plymouth, UK.

More information about this series at
https://link.springer.com/bookseries/16540

Jeremy Woodcock

Families and Individuals Living with Trauma

A Guide for Therapists, Relatives, and Friends

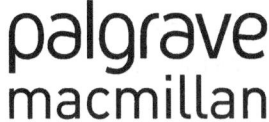

Jeremy Woodcock
Nailsworth, UK

ISSN 2662-9127   ISSN 2662-9135   (electronic)
Palgrave Texts in Counselling and Psychotherapy
ISBN 978-3-030-79038-7   ISBN 978-3-030-79039-4   (eBook)
https://doi.org/10.1007/978-3-030-79039-4

Cover illustration: Tatiana Gerich/Alamy Stock Photo

This Palgrave Macmillan imprint is published by the registered company Springer Nature Switzerland AG
The registered company address is: Gewerbestrasse 11, 6330 Cham, Switzerland

Acknowledgments

This book has emerged out of years of many years of work at The Medical Foundation, now Freedom from Torture, in London and I am deeply indebted to my many colleagues there for discussions, arguments, warm friendship, opportunities for co-work, and team experience. The people who come to mind are Abood Tuma, Alex Sklan, Anne-Marie Fox, Annie Ellison, Barbara Dearnley, Caroline Gorst-Unsworth, Dick Blackwell, Derek Summerfield, Funda Kansu, Gill Hinshelwood, Gillian Ballance, Helen Bamber, Irene Aitman, Jane Shackman, Jeanette Campbell-Johnston, John Schlapobersky, Karen Callaghan, Mesfin Demissie, Naomi Richman, Nagul Subramaniam, Nimisha Patel, Perico Rodrigues, Richard McKane, Sally Verity-Smith, Seda Sengun, Sheila Melzak, Susan Levy and Zohreh Rahimi. In addition I wish to thank my teachers, supervisors, and psychotherapy colleagues in London and the South West and beyond including Arul Maria Arokiasamy, Ann Miller, Annette Mendelsohn, Barry Mason, Biddy Arnott, my many colleagues in Sweden at Krisochtraumaenheten, and at Gloucestershire Action for Refugees and Asylum Seekers, David Jones, David Pocock, Elsa Jones, Jane Cutler, John Byng-Hall, Judith Lask,

Judy Ryde, Kedar Dwivedi, Lennox Thomas, Marita Eastmond, Nigel Wellings, Mark Rivett, Philip Darley, Sally Box, Tim Hockridge and Tony Navin. Something of work with all these colleagues has rubbed off on me in ways that have been deepening, enjoyable, and challenging in equal measure. Finally to Arlene Vetere for her patience and gentle guidance, to Rudi Dallos for being a critical friend, and to the skill of colleagues at Palgrave in bringing this book to birth.

About This Book

This book is a book for you if you are a survivor of trauma, or if someone you love, a family member, or friend has survived a serious trauma. It sets out to explain trauma and describes pathways through and out the other side. For survivors it shows how you can recover, and for family and friends it shows how to support and help. For therapists working with individuals and families it sets out to be an essential text, describing how trauma affects us, and it reveals in detail what works therapeutically, and how to apply these ideas in practice.

Contents

List of Figures

List of Tables

1

Introduction

If someone you love, a family member or friend has suffered a serious
trauma, this is a book for you. It is a book for the general reader and
it is a book for therapists. It sets out to explain trauma, describes a way
through it, and how you can support and help. If you are a therapist
working with individuals and families it sets out to be an essential text.
It reveals in detail what works therapeutically and how to navigate a way
through. Each chapter takes a theme such as beginnings, or body brain
and trauma, or when disaster strikes and with stories of the work and
case material describes what can be learned in order to be a supportive
family member and friend, or an effective therapist. There is naturally
an inevitable tension between being either a family member, friend, or
therapist and how much one can do to help. This is not a book about
encouraging family members and friends to be therapists, but what it
attempts is to describe clearly what can be supportive, and then charts in
more depth the nature of therapeutic work that will help. By describing
the deeper therapeutic work it endeavors to create an understanding
of what work with trauma entails, and to deepen family members and
friends capacity to live alongside someone else's trauma in ways that

© The Author(s), under exclusive license to Springer Nature
Switzerland AG 2022
J. Woodcock, *Families and Individuals Living with Trauma,*
Palgrave Texts in Counselling and Psychotherapy,
https://doi.org/10.1007/978-3-030-79039-4_1

are deeply informed and compassionate. This goes to the heart of why this book has been written. My experience of work with trauma over thirty years is that when trauma strikes it doesn't just affect individuals, it resonates through family and friendship groups, and across communities. Trauma tears holes in the fabric of lives, and here are descriptions of how this can be lived with and repaired; not just reassembled and put together again but opened up into a place where we have a deeper sense of connection with ourselves and each other.

The word trauma is used liberally and uncritically throughout the book although in my professional work I take a far more critical stance in relation to its use, and this raises very important issues to do with how we survive the bad things that happen to us. Extreme events happen frequently but not everyone who endures such an event will suffer psychological trauma. The reasons for this are complex and can be understood in terms of hardiness and resilience. This can involve many factors from how we process emotional overload neurologically and physically, through to the nature of the communities in which we live, and most importantly the social meanings that are ascribed to extreme events. This doesn't mean that trauma only appears when it is labeled as such. Trauma can live underground for years, consider the *Me Too* movement; or generations, consider *Black Lives Matter*, or centuries, consider the pernicious effects of slavery. My preference is to use extreme events to label the event itself, and trauma as the psychological aftermath that may follow, but is not inevitable. In the territory that lies between there are a plethora of contending forces: how much light and voice that are brought to events to validate experience; how much support is forthcoming; the extent to which people are empowered to cope with events, and in the extreme moment how overwhelmed we are in ways that compel us to respond in ways that undo us. To this can be added our individual capacity for hardiness or our vulnerability to overwhelm, and these are not static qualities but are deeply influenced by social factors, the quality of our relationships and quite critically, our fluctuating capacity for reflection. However, in the book trauma is used liberally for those who self-identify as being traumatized, and for families, friends, and therapists who would offer this description. In brief, this means people who have survived extreme circumstances that would ordinarily overwhelm any of us, and who have emerged in various ways emotionally altered by what they have endured. This is a book for them.

This is also a book that sits within the traditions of family therapy. This liberating way of viewing the world and the relationships within which we live and that live through us underpins the writing. What may disappoint systemic family therapists is that systemic phrases are not used as a great deal. However, those ideas are threaded throughout the text, richly integrated with the many traditions that have grappled with trauma. It seems an absolute given that when someone is affected by a trauma this is not merely an individual thing but will resonate in a circular way through family, friendships, intimate relationships and back and forth through the community in which they live. It is the gift of family therapy to understand very deeply how this happens. Even more importantly family therapists have the courage, and no doubt the compulsion and conviction to engage with individuals in the contexts of their family's and to borrow a phrase, to engage with the contexts of family's in individuals. Furthermore, the critical voice that family therapy brings to therapeutic work, by which is meant its liberating capacity to see symptoms of distress as not residing merely in individuals but as a shared experience will be found here, as well as the impulse to meet survivors and their families and friends through the habits of their own self-descriptions not through the lens of pathology.

Over years of work with psychological trauma what becomes clear is that trauma cannot be owned by any one particular brand of psychotherapy, it is too complex, too protean to be captured in the folds of any one tradition. Indeed this much is tellingly true, that trauma as a category of human experience is also created and shaped by psychological descriptions and its interventions. This places a burden on psychotherapists to hold our knowledge and experience lightly, to share, and to borrow ideas, and this book is full of both sharing and borrowings. The other aspect of this is that trauma as a human experience is held in the folds of other traditions. Extreme events and trauma run through in literature from the earliest times. Draupadi, the fascinating fiery heroine of the Indian epic the Mahabharata journeys from pitiless tragedy to transcendent glory; Achilles is undone by the death of Patroclus under the walls of Troy; Wen-siang (1995) who gave poetic voice to tragic experience as the Mongol Horde swept across the Central Asian steppes; the weighted encounter of Ibn al-Arabi with Averroës and exile from Spain that his life and writing transcended; the tragic unfolding of Iréne Némirovsky's *Suite Française* (2007): the limpid poetry of exile of Pablo Neruda; the agonized cry of pain from Wole Soyinka's *The Man Died* (1972).

What emerges from these reflections is that trauma has shaped human existence from time immemorial, and that our responses to it cannot be merely psychological. We find it decorating pottery unearthed in Attica, in monuments to fallen across the world, in the barbed wire that divides continents. What this propels us toward is the realization that because of its propensity to divide and shame and silence trauma needs its witnesses, and it should only be left in a private space at the choosing of survivors. This means that those who work in the semi-private domain of psychotherapy will be helped by partnership with witnesses outside the consulting room. There are delicate choices to be made here, for instance whether to join the march, or to write, or paint or compose or perform, or to support those that do. One of the wonderful realizations in the systemic world view is that these different perspectives are joined up at multiple levels of context. One of the tasks of therapy, when contexts are hidden from each other, is to uncover them, sometimes with the delicate patience of an archaeologist, sometimes with the explosive exuberance of performance.

You will find many omissions and mistakes in this book. There is little about intergenerational trauma, although the hope is that in giving a voice to the inner and outer aspects of extreme experience, that the chain of transmission will be broken. There is little included from the Jungian oeuvre, although there is a great deal from that tradition that speaks to trauma particularly as it brings together body work and its wide-ranging understanding of archetypal contexts: the work of Marion Woodman (2005) comes to mind. There is little of the Cognitive Behavioral tradition, although its work slides through and is honored by its presence in many dimensions, for instance within EMDR, and through mindfulness. There is also little of the Intersubjective tradition although its practices deeply inform the relational nature of much of the work described. There is also little written explicitly of race and culture nor of difference, nor of gender and power, although themes from these are picked up in work described, and the hope is that these will somewhat inform how we can stand in solidarity with experiences shaped from within those perspectives, and propel us into wanting to learn more. Trauma can dispossess us, and undoubtedly falls unevenly on those with least power and voice, I would only want that the emotional understanding embodied in this book brings power to those who have suffered, and to their families, their friends, their communities, and their therapists.

Finally, an important part of this book is that at the end of each chapter there are a set of questions and reflections. These are for families, friends, and survivors to consider together in your family, support, and friendship circle. They are an invitation to use the challenge of trauma, which can do so much to separate us, as an opportunity for reflection, connection, and transformation. These are also ideas therapists may hold in mind when working with families and individuals.

References

Némirovsky, Iréne. 2007. *Suite Française*. London: Vintage.
Soyinka, Wole. 1972. *The Man Died*. London: Arrow Press.
Wen-siang. 1995. *Sleepless Nights: Verses for the Wakeful*, trans. Thomas Cleary. Berkeley: North Atlantic Books.
Woodman, Marion. 2005. Body and Soul: Honoring Marion Woodman. In *Spring: A Journal of Archetype and Culture*. New York: Springer.

2

Beginnings

If you, or someone you love, or someone you work with professionally has suffered a trauma this book seeks to take everything that flows out of that experience in a way that makes it understandable, and to create the possibility of healing. Chapter by chapter we consider different aspects of trauma, how they effect individuals and families, and over the course of the book we chart a journey through the effects of trauma and out the other side.

Consider Max, at 26 after years of being confined in apprenticeships in the catering industry he broke out and traveled alone to the Middle East. There he was befriended by a similarly aged young man who invited him to visit his village in the remote north of the country. After several days of travel by coach there were signs of a huge military presence, they began to pass through army checkpoints. Max was reassured by his companion that this was quite normal but their anxiety grew as the build up of troops and armored vehicles escalated. Eventually at a checkpoint deep in the region the passengers were ordered off the bus. Max was separated and questioned and taken over the hills to an army command post. His entreaties that he was merely a curious traveler were dismissed. He

© The Author(s), under exclusive license to Springer Nature
Switzerland AG 2022
J. Woodcock, *Families and Individuals Living with Trauma*,
Palgrave Texts in Counselling and Psychotherapy,
https://doi.org/10.1007/978-3-030-79039-4_2

was interrogated over several days by an English-speaking army captain who didn't appear to believe his story and said, "Tourists don't travel out here, it's too dangerous." He was accused of being a spy, and told, "Tell us the truth, or we just might kill you. There are many rebel groups fighting in this area. You could just disappear, no one would know." He was completely terrified and told me, "In those moments I had never felt so alone in my whole life. Everyone I had ever loved just disappeared from my mind. My mum to whom I was so close was no longer there for me. I was completely, utterly, terrifyingly alone."

After he was released and once he was physically safe Max left the country as soon as he could. He didn't dare fly out because he was terrified of the authorities and so he traveled overland. It was only when he crossed into the neighboring country and reported to his consulate that he felt he could tell his story and that he felt believed, and they helped to repatriate him.

When Max got back home, despite his wish that it was otherwise, he felt completely alienated from his family and friends. He said they seemed to understand in a way, but they didn't really get it. No one really connected to the depth and seriousness of his terror. He said it felt like the loving part of him, the very center out of which he loved and felt lived had been swallowed up.

It was striking what a tender and thoughtful young man Max was. He came over as deeply thoughtful and loving, and yet he couldn't connect and relate those feelings to his loved ones. They felt cool and distant to him, and he was deeply perplexed and disturbed by this change in himself. He also found that he panicked very easily, and he said his sleep was interrupted by horrible dreams, and sometimes though more rarely, he found himself in daydream-like states where he felt that he was back in detention being interrogated again. He sort of understood these affects on himself and was able to relate them quite perceptively to different aspects of what had happened to him but he was disturbed by their persistence and energy, and the fact that no amount of thinking about it relieved what he was experiencing and how he felt.

We can understand what was happening to Max after he got home if we look at each aspect of his experience in turn. Ultimately it isn't helpful to divide body and mind when thinking about trauma but because so many of us are so deeply schooled by our Western sensibility into thinking and experiencing the world as divided it will help if we begin from there and add a third area giving us a three-part division, body, mind, and environment.

Bodily Signs and Symptoms

Max suffered from fear, panic, breathlessness, anxiety, he was easily startled, had difficulty falling asleep, and he woke easily.

Mental Signs and Symptoms

Max had frightening dreams at night, and during the day he had deep, gripping recollections of being back in detention. With awful regret and sadness he found that he had lost his loving feelings, and he felt alienated and very much alone.

Environment Signs and Symptoms

Max panicked in dark corridors, he had a strong dislike of noise and bustle, and disliked loud or sudden noises from vehicles. He had a deep sense of feeling separate from life around him, sometimes it felt like life was "through there" on the other side of the bubble he found himself in.

Making a Story of Trauma

Don't rush someone who has been through an extreme experience into telling their story; show you are interested but wait for them. Even if you are a close family member and know them really well, allow trust to develop that you can be a safe person who can really hear what has happened. There may be shocking and shameful things that aren't easily revealed; the story may also come out in broken, disjointed, and fragmentary ways. Allow for blank and missing portions, probe a little but don't push too hard; try to co-construct what you are being told, in other words make sense of it together. Ask simple open clarifying questions that leave them in charge of the telling. Don't be tempted to wrap it up and make sense of it too soon, allow it to be tentative and emergent.

Guidancecoercive—Open questions

Open questions need more than a "yes" or "no" to answer them	Why didn't you get off then?
	How did it seem to you?
Open questions often begin with a how, what, or why	What did you do?
How come you chose that route?	Why was that suggested?
What happened next?	Open questions encourage conversation, often I'll ask, "Is there more?" Or, "Tell me more"

Very often when someone has been through an extreme experience they may not want to talk at all at first. Very often what they need is to know that all the practicalities of their life are in place. Helping them with all that is the best place to start. This may include medical attention as well as sorting out issues with accommodation and work. Once these are in place they may want to open up but don't rush.

Key Point—Attend to the Practicalities

Often it is the practical things that are at the top of peoples list of priorities when they have been through a trauma; do they have enough money, a place to stay, can there medical needs be met.

There is good evidence that some people emotionally digest traumatic events in their own way and never need to seek much help outside themselves. There is also evidence that if people are pressed to recall what happened too quickly, before they feel the need, that fragments of what happened get embedded in their memories in ways that are unhelpful, but when left to their own devices they process the experience and make sense of it in there own way, and the awfulness of it just simply flows away into the past. As a rule, if someone is preoccupied by what happened, if it really has them in its grip several months after the events, then they probably need to talk, and as we will learn in the chapters that follow, not only to talk but process what has happened physically and emotionally.

Max wanted to tell me his story. I wasn't necessarily keen to push him to reveal everything in a hurry but he trusted the process and was eager to get on, so we pieced it together and tried to understand what particular aspects of his symptoms might have been linked to what he had been through. In doing this his story took on an almost "four dimensional" feel.

The Four Dimensions of the Trauma Story

1. A story that makes sense in time as a simple narrative a follows b follows c.
2. A story that links the physical and emotional aspects (He slapped me hard in the face, my cheeks stung and I felt angry, frightened, and ashamed).
3. A story that makes sense of one's inner thoughts, feelings, and one's intrinsic sense of self (I had always thought of myself as easy going and sociable and now I am unusually introverted).
4. A trauma story will often have a mythic "out of time" quality (I look back on it now and it seems like a dream; I had always thought of those halcyon blue skies as full of hope and promise of a bright year ahead and now they seem raw and pitiless; there are moments when I'm not sure if I am awake, or dreaming, or imagining things).

Each of these dimensions overlaps and influences each other and while it is important to be factual it is also important to allow space for the emotional and mythic aspects of the trauma.

Key Point—Trauma can be a life changing event and it will have deeply emotional and mythic qualities to it, these need to be given space and understanding. Sometimes myths, and stories, music, song, drama, poetry, television, art work, religious beliefs, and other forms of belief and expression will play a part in understanding and digesting trauma.

Trust

One of the fundamental things that can be damaged by a traumatic experience is what has been described as "basic trust". Basic trust is our sense that the world, and at best, our family and friends are safe, and that life is predictable. After trauma this sense of basic trust can be absent and we are likely to trust people much less easily and be more wary in new situations. Because of this we cannot assume that a person who has been traumatized is going to automatically trust us. Trust has to be carefully earned. Max was not surprised that he trusted the world less easily, he knew it had let him down, and he reckoned he had been foolish, in some ways, to have so easily trusted the situation he got into while abroad. However, he was really disconcerted that he no longer trusted his mother, she had been his absolutely dependable rock throughout his life. This change in how we experience significant emotional bonds is a key experience for some people who have experienced extreme events and we will consider in greater depth how this happens later on.

> **Key Point—Basic Trust**
>
> Basic trust is the sense that we live in a predictable world, that life will not surprise us or let us down, that we can generally trust other people, that we are lovable and we can love.

Making Sense of Signs and Symptoms

Common sense helps a lot when we have been traumatized. Common sense can give a broad brush stroke explanation of what has happened, it can also be the simple explanation that makes most sense to our family and friends. However, for many people who have been through an extreme event a simple explanation may not be enough partly because it doesn't explain the psychological symptoms that follow. Common psychological symptoms may include:

Signs of Being More Easily Aroused

- Irritability and anger.
- Being easily triggered and startled.
- Being hyper alert.
- Loss of concentration.
- Poor sleep—finding it hard to drop off and waking during the night.

Avoiding Things to Do with the Trauma and Being Less Involved in Life

- Avoiding thoughts and feelings and conversations associated with the trauma.
- Avoiding activities, places, or people that bring memories of the trauma

- Not being able to remember important details of the trauma.
- A decreased interest in activities that were previously important.
- Feelings of indifference or distance from others.
- Having a narrower range of feelings. For example struggling to feel joy, or to take pleasure in things, or to have loving feelings.
- Having less sense of a future, as if career, children, or a normal life span will not happen or no longer matter.

Having a Sense That the Extreme Event Is Ever Present

- Having repeated distressing, intrusive memories of the event, this may include momentary images, half-thoughts and bodily sensations.
- Repeatedly having distressing dreams.
- Acting or feeling as if the traumatic event is happening again. This may include a sense of reliving the experience, as well as hallucinations and flashbacks.
- Intense feelings of distress when coming up against things that have characteristics of the traumatic event.

This template of signs and symptoms is taken from the diagnostic guidelines of the American Psychiatric Association (2013). It includes some symptoms that are seemingly in conflict with each other such as being easily stirred up or aroused, versus trying to avoid thoughts and feelings versus a sense of the trauma always being present. These are the tensions and inner conflicts of trauma that can make it confusing. We try to avoid the traumatic memory, but we're on a knife edge. High arousal and panic is kicked off by the limbic system, it brings thoughts into our mind, and then freezes them out. We rock back and forth, and we might wish there was a drug we could take that would calm us down and sort it all out, but there isn't. The chapters in front of us explain all these things and the ways out.

Often Trauma Comes Out Sideways

Sometimes trauma may revisit in panic attacks, palpitations, being wired up, being easily triggered, being fearful of dangers that don't worry other people, believing that one's life is going to end, spending much of life in a panicky state. Sometimes it may show itself in hidden ways by depression and a loss of interest in life, or by use of alcohol and drugs and driving addictive behaviors to numb feelings out. These are the wild ways that trauma can come out sideways.

The Wish to Remember and the Need to Forget

If we think about Max the most distressing experience for him once he got home was that he felt estranged from his friends and in particular his mother. But on the other hand he was grateful to be left in his withdrawn state of mind by everyone. He didn't want his memories stirred up because he found that they made him really distressed. It felt like no one could help him when he got into that frame of mind. On the other hand his friends and his mother were worried because they knew he was sleeping badly and had nightmares. He felt upset by these but he didn't want to talk about them because it didn't feel safe. This was the bind he was in when we met.

Key Point

Systemic Scaffolding

The web of relationships with family, friends, community; work and leisure activities; the things that give sense to our life, such as arts and crafts, and the natural world; our histories, and beliefs and ethics. The capacity to evaluate the scaffold, to reflect on it and make use of it in a reciprocal way.

Family and friends can provide and support the systemic scaffolding by exploring what makes up the scaffolding for a survivor—family,

---

friends, community contacts, home, work, life routines, leisure activities and interests, and working out how much of that feels useful and dependable this side of surviving an extreme experience, and how things can be adapted to make things work more positively on their behalf. For example, a young woman who had been through a terrifying ordeal couldn't drive her car afterwards, so friends were recruited to drive her places. After his trauma and young man found it very difficult to sleep alone, he lived temporarily with his parents and later friends stayed over with him at his place until he had recovered. A man couldn't work his regular hours after his sickness period came to an end so negotiations with his employer enabled him to work a more flexible work routine that took account of his vulnerability until he had recovered.

Key Point—The Wish to Remember and the Need to Forget

Trauma has some symptoms that seem to be in conflict such as being easily stirred up or aroused, versus trying to avoid thoughts and feelings versus a sense of the trauma always being present. This conflict has been summed up as, "the wish to remember and the need to forget."

A Systemic Scaffolding

We have the inner experience of our lives and around it we have what can be described as a systemic scaffolding, this is the external structures that hold us together. The systemic scaffolding consists of relationships with family and friends and community; the things that employ us during the day such as work, caring for others and the endeavors that make sense of our lives. It will also include the wider world that creates the contexts in which we lead our lives, the worlds of community, politics, arts and crafts, as well as the local, national, and international environment.

Extreme events can make a massive impact on the systemic scaffolding: family members, and friends and community members can be injured or killed; our work and employment and interests may be compromised or we may not feel the wish to continue with them; our world may not feel very safe anymore, and it may actually be objectively unsafe; the political situation around us and conditions in the wider world may not be supportive, and may even be hostile.

Whatever the case, when someone has been through extreme events it helps to put the scaffolding in place, practically as described above or to make an inventory that describes and acknowledges what has been compromised and what can be put back in its place. For Max the systemic scaffolding consisted of his mum, her community, and his friends. In the wider world he was troubled how his adventure had turned into a personal disaster for him and how familiar holiday destinations that he had always trusted no longer felt safe. His work was also a struggle—it had always been a place that was demanded hard work, but he had been dependable and valued. Now he struggled after nights when he slept poorly, his concentration wasn't good, he was distracted by personal preoccupations in the fast-moving kitchen where he worked, and he was sometimes really freaked out by the noisy demanding atmosphere.

Working together we put together an inventory of what worked and what didn't hold up for him in his systemic scaffolding. It looked something like this:

- His mum was dependable: but he felt estranged.
- His mum's friends were good people; but he didn't want to open up to them now much beyond the superficial.
- Work was reliable: but he felt unreliable and he worried their patience would fail.
- His home and immediate environment felt safe: the wider world didn't feel safe at all.

Beginning at the Beginning

The scaffolding is a good place to begin when we are considering how to proceed with supporting someone with a trauma and to see if they would benefit from therapeutic work. If someone has a decent scaffolding around them supporting them and working through a trauma will usually be much more straightforward. However, we can see from Max's experience that the scaffolding is not merely an objective state of affairs, it has a deeply subjective character. Max understood that how he felt and responded to things could be weighed up and debated and a middle ground might be found. Not everyone has such a clear supporting scaffolding nor as much reflective capacity.

Weighing up how good their scaffolding is with them can help you and them decide if they are ready to do therapeutic work with their trauma. We can characterize how ready a person may be to work with their trauma using the framework below that is a mix of how good their scaffolding is and their capacity for reflection.

Capacity for Reflection

It has to be borne in mind that our capacity for reflection varies. When we are under stress our capacity for reflection can narrow in scope and lose its resilience, we can become more tunnel-like, more preoccupied, less flexible, more concrete, and absolute in our thinking. This means that when someone is practically and emotionally supported their thinking can relax and expand, and their capacity for reflection may deepen. This means the categories above need to be seen on a continuum, they are not fixed, and people's sense of their scaffolding and their capacity for reflection will vary over time.

Guidance

Capacity for Reflection

They have experienced trauma and have a good dependable scaffolding around them—relationships, employment and living circumstances are stable	Have a good capacity for reflection	May be ready for therapeutic help
They have trauma and do not have a good dependable scaffolding around them but they have a decent capacity for reflection	Have a good capacity for reflection	May be ready for therapeutic help but will need more scaffolding
They have experienced trauma and have a good dependable scaffolding around them—relationships, employment and living circumstances are stable	Are not reflective or psychologically minded	May not respond to pure therapeutic help; may benefit from support that blends therapeutic insight and practical and emotional support

Supporting Someone Who Doesn't Want Therapeutic Help

Not everyone wants therapy, or is ready for it. Supporting them requires using good listening skills, being emotionally and practically supportive, opening up issues but letting them decide. It requires good listening skills and a capacity to be supportive, to help them in very practical ways with the scaffolding.

Supporting someone practically and emotionally may go on for many months. They may emerge from the trauma in their own good time or they may eventually seek therapeutic help. Being supportive in a way that is respectful and led by them can only help.

Felt Experience

One of the things that was central to the therapeutic work Max did can be described as Max's "felt experience," this is quite a subtle idea but once grasped it can deepen our appreciation of life. These ideas are suggested for therapists to adopt in their work with survivors. It is probably out of being confronted by the profound depths of felt experience that people who have been through extreme experiences emerge with a deeper appreciation of the holistic qualities of life and relationships.

The American philosopher Eugene Gendlin (1996) struck the term "felt experience" to describe the vague bodily awareness that our body speaks truths to us if we can attune to these subtle inner processes and listen with the inner ear. Working with the therapist Carl Rogers he developed felt experience and felt shift as powerful ways to self-understanding. It is a ground breaking idea that so closely matches common sense that we can easily overlook its subtleties. It means paying careful attention to the sensations that arise in us, not naming them or labeling them as good or bad but just dwelling on the sensations long enough so an appreciation of them emerges and not making a great distinction between emotions we can identify and name and other bodily sensations. When we pay bare attention like this to what arises in us and allow our attention to focus a clear sense of felt experience emerges. If we stay with that felt experience another process emerges that they described as a "felt shift". It's like this, imagine you have had a sense of unease, stay with that sense of unease, don't describe it in words, merely track how it feels in various places as you scan your body. You notice a tightness in the neck, a sense of feeling slightly sick; your impulse is to back off, to push the experience out of your mind and body; instead stay focused, allow a clearer resolution of the sensations to emerge.

Guidance

Listening Skills

1. Face the speaker and hold eye contact

2. Be relaxed and attentive, be present, pay attention, be ready to serve

3. Keep an open mind, don't judge or jump to conclusions

4. Try and picture what is being said

5. Don't interrupt

6. Don't offer solutions—just listen

7. Wait for them to pause before asking open clarifying questions

8. Try to feel what the speaker is feeling

9. Give feedback, nodding, affirming the feelings and words of what's been said if these are clear

10. Tune in to the non-verbal, words are only part of he message

---

Felt Shift

If we stay with these sensations Gendlin reckons a felt shift will emerge, a sense of excitement, of discovery and optimism. Of course it may not always be like this, perhaps a darker set of sensations may emerge; but stay with these and a deeper appreciation of your capacity to stay with more challenging feelings will emerge. Felt shift often has hints of profound emergent understanding, courage, and resolution. For instance, a man focuses on how angry he is with his father and finds it very uncomfortable to admit to those emotions. He says, "I really don't want to go there" but gently encouraged he then says, "I don't want to admit it but I feel like murdering him, it's so strong, it's horrible." He is both encouraged to stay with it, but simultaneously given explicit permission to stop if he feels overwhelmed; the latitude of this holding stance by the therapist enables him to feel emotionally contained and he sticks with it, and as he focuses and breathes into the sensations that emerge he says, "Not only do I feel almost intolerably angry but I also feel deep tenderness, we were both trapped, I feel things as if I were a child and I see and feel things as though I were in my fathers skin."

An approach that can guide therapists and families through powerful and conflicting emotions members is felt sense, indeed felt sense can guide us through the most gentle and subtle emotions as well. Felt sense was developed by the American philosopher Eugene Gendlin, it is a ground breaking idea that so closely matches common sense that we can easily overlook its subtleties. In essence felt sense is a way to map our internal bodily awareness of our sensations and emotions. We can become more deeply aware and attuned to these when we use an exercise that Gendlin calls focusing. The method is as follows: we are invited to pause and register any bodily sensations and emotions within ourselves; we dwell on these while not making a great distinction between emotions we can identify and name and other bodily sensations that may be the precursors of emotions or merely simple bodily sensations. We are asked to make no judgment about our experience, but just to locate feelings and sensations, to properly register them and dwell on them. As we focus their qualities reveal themselves more fully. Gendlin says, ultimately when we focus we almost certainly will experience what he describes as a "felt shift", that is the sensations and emotions that we think of as familiar give way and more profound insights emerge. For instance, a man focuses on how angry he is with his father and finds it very uncomfortable to admit to those emotions. He says, "I really don't want to go there" but gently encouraged he then says, "I don't want to admit it but I feel like murdering him, it's so strong, it's horrible." He is both encouraged to stay with it, but simultaneously given explicit permission to stop if he feels overwhelmed; the latitude of this holding stance by the therapist enables him to feel emotionally contained and he sticks with it, and as he focuses and breathes into the sensations that emerge he says, "Not only do I feel almost intolerably angry but I also feel deep tenderness, we were both trapped, I feel things as if I were a child and I see and feel things as though I were in my fathers skin."

When someone has experienced an extreme event it may be very troubling for them to stay felt sense and with bodily experience. The skill of this work is helping them to do that, taking a small part of their experience and staying with that while something opens up, and a shift occurs. It is also important that as someone helping you can appreciate felt sense, focusing, and felt shift and the lighter and darker parts of your experience which that entails.

Exercise

Felt Sense and Felt ShiftExercise for Therapists and Survivor
  Bring an experience to mind
  Scan your body for your felt sensations
  Focus on those felt bodily sensations however vague
  Stay with them as they resolve and clarify—don't name them, or label them good or bad, try and stay with the sensations paying them "bare attention"
  Just allow whatever happens to happen, ease your way into a deeper appreciation of what is beginning to emerge, this may be a felt shift
  What does this felt shift allow and signify—stay with this as interpretation emerges

---

Finding the Middle Ground

It is really important to find the middle ground when supporting someone after a trauma and when doing therapeutic work. The middle ground is that place where things may feel uneasy but things are bearable, they can be remembered, brought into mind and understood. It is closely related to what is described as the window of tolerance, the space between what is bearable and what is unbearable. As one works in that zone the middle ground expands, so more things can be tolerated and understood. For Max the middle ground looked like this: work and home and close relationships were dependable but he felt those relationships had changed in ways that were to do with him and his experience and were intrinsically nothing to do with his mother and friends. Like a great deal of work with trauma our work began in that middle ground exploring his felt experiences, working with his recollections of the terror, and gradually his tolerance and understanding of what he had endured expanded. We worked together, over the course of a number of months and Max began to feel better and felt restored to his family and friends. We will explore this sort of work in greater detail in later chapters.

Guidance

The Middle Ground and the Window of Tolerance

The middle ground is the emotional space we occupy that is easy, it encompasses what may be difficult but not the stuff that is distinctly scary or unbearable to bring into mind: that is the stuff that is captured by work with the window of tolerance

The window of tolerance is a more precise term that defines the precise edge that marks the boundary between what is comfortable and can be brought into mind and spoken about and what is intensely uncomfortable

When exploring the window of tolerance it is very important be led by the survivor. Ask them to signal very clearly when conversation is straying over the edge into what is unbearable. Look carefully yourself for signs that things are uncomfortable and with their agreement return into the zone of what is comfortable. Work with their place of safety, use an agreed distraction method, use breathing and relaxation and take time before waiting their signal that they are ready to explore across the edge of the window of tolerance again

Therapeutic work aims to expand the window of tolerance gradually over time so that eventually everything can be brought into mind

---

In the chapters that follow we will look at each of the aspects described in this chapter in more detail and understand how individuals and families can have their well-being restored. It is written to help you to take hold of what is happening either to you, or to someone you care about and to suggest what may help and guide you through a process of healing. Most importantly this book is intended to help you as an individual or family understand and work through your trauma making use of the wealth of your own resources, if that is your wish and to help you work effectively with the good sources of therapeutic help that are out there. Furthermore, it is intended as a guide for therapists to work along side the resources that are so richly part of individuals and families who have survived extreme events.

What We Can Do as Family and Friends

Consider all this together with the survivor and in your family/friendship circle, take turns to speak, listen, and reflect.

Listen and tune in to the survivor's story, follow their lead, don't push, make sense of it together with them, tolerate gaps that are there, it may not make sense at first, just be as open hearted and open minded as you can.

Understand how trauma affects a survivor and how a survivor may act and behave; there's no template, everyone is different, but the signs and symptoms at the beginning of this chapter offer a starting point. Understand how trust may be hard.

Listen with an open mind, be non-judgmental.

Ask open questions

Anticipate how this trauma might resonate through the family/friendship network. Maybe put this as a simple question in the family/friendship circle, and without anyone butting in sit back listen to each others ideas.

Consider the systemic scaffolding that the survivor may need, think with them how best to support.

Focus on practicalities that the survivor requires.

Understand the window of tolerance, work out together with them what the survivor can bear to open up, and what they want to avoid right now, be led by them.

Be a reflective support, take time to focus on your inner lives find your supportive circle and to be reflective with them.

References

American Psychiatric Association. 2013. *Diagnostic and Statistical Manual of Mental Disorders*, 5th ed. Washington, DC: APA.

Gendlin, Eugene. 1996. *Focusing-Oriented Psychotherapy: A Manual of the Experiential Method*. London: Guilford Press.

3

Body, Brain and Trauma

Emotional attachment is hugely important in trauma. Attachment is a profound human process, not only a human process but a profound animal process that shapes our physiology and mentality and our very being in the world from the beginning of our life. One of the mantras of the attachment expert Pat Crittenden is that "children seek safety" (2008). Seeking safety is a simple yet sophisticated process that highlights the physiological drive toward attachment.

In the 1930s the Austrian scientist Konrad Lorenz observed that Greylag geese that saw him immediately after they hatched responded to him as if he were their mother. This imprinting, as Lorenz called it, is a fundamental physiological sign of the attachment drive, the drive toward safety that is present in all mammals. Naturally it is more complex in humans who take longer to develop after birth but very similar processes

J. Woodcock, *Families and Individuals Living with Trauma*, Palgrave Texts in Counselling and Psychotherapy, https://doi.org/10.1007/978-3-030-79039-4_3

are there in all of us. For instance, infants are soothed in the arms of their mothers in a two-way mother and child bond in which mother offers safety and baby responds so completely it can be observed that their biologies actually intertwine as their bodily states attune to each other. Mother's breath and heart beat slow down, her alertness settles into a relaxed middle ground where she is mostly focused on her baby but is also open to cues that need her response in the immediate environment. Similarly baby falls into an optimum middle ground between being wakefully alert, perhaps with hunger or discomfort of some sort, and sleep. This intertwining of mother and baby's biologies can be tracked by the hormones that ebb and flow through their bodies and brains. Research by scientists and clinicians such as Alan Sroufe (1996), and Allan Schore et al. (2021) that have followed the attachments of people from infancy into mid-life show that the quality of care that a mother gives to her infant child shapes its capacity to relate to others in later life, and crucially also shapes its resilience to stress. What was noticed time and again in all the studies that these authors cite was that the mother's capacity to attune to her infants needs in a balanced way that matched their infants needs by neither being intrusive nor too laid back and neglectful later produced adults who could meet stress by neither being over excited or unresponsive.

Basic Trust

What came over very clearly was that the key to growing up well was how mothers felt about their children and the nature of the give and take relationship between them. Parents who were warm and responsive to their children's needs, and who felt instinctively protective toward them created children and adults who were not only emotionally secure but also resilient to the ordinary challenges of life. This state of affairs can be summarized by what people working in this field for many years have described as basic trust. The neuroscience of basic trust is outlined in the box below. It is important for us to understand that basic trust is not a fixed thing, it has many layers that interact and influence each other; neurobiology, relationships and the environment each plays its part.

Learning Point

Basic Trust

The neuropeptide oxytocin released by the mother at birth stimulates the bond with her baby, in particular it creates a sensitivity to the child's unique smell and opens up neural pathways that imprints the child's distinctive signals, sounds, and cries within the key emotional circuits in the mother's brain.

Oxytocin has been described as the cuddle hormone, it supports the mother's instinctive desire to be responsive to her child.

Serotonin floods through the body and calms and lowers irritability.

Mirror neurones in mother and child's frontal cortex, linked to the limbic system, enable them to "read" each other's intentions and enables the mother to accurately attune to her baby's emotional state.

Baby experiences the world as responsive and dependable: a model of environment and relationships is created in the baby's body-mind that is safe, dependable, and trustworthy.

It is this basic trust that can be shattered by traumatic experience. Indeed, when a shocking trauma is experienced what makes it traumatic is not exactly the experience itself but the manner in which the experience attacks and changes our fundamental relationship to basic trust. This goes some way to explain why some people are deeply affected by trauma and others escape deeply challenging experiences much more easily. In what follows we will peel apart the layers of attachment, neurobiology, and basic trust more deeply.

The Limbic System: Our Fight and Flight and Freeze Protector

The limbic system has been described as the body's early warning system, alerting us to danger. It is our fight and flight protector, looking after us in danger. However, it is a great deal more than that, it is the fundamental part of our psycho-biology that maintains our awareness, and our sense of being in the world through our five sense organs, sight, hearing, smell, taste, and touch at an optimal level. Indeed, in an almost uncanny way it goes beyond our five sense organs because it is also attuned to be responsive to proprioception—that is our sense of where our bodies are in space. For instance, the limbic system provides the synthesis of our sense organs that tells us as we lean out to stroke the cat that he will be there just slinking under our outstretched finger tips, or as we sit back in our dining chair that the chair will be there right under us, or as we run down a trail that our feet will fall in the right place on its twisting surfaces. Furthermore, the limbic system is uncanny in its ability to alert us to danger even before our conscious mind has registered the risk to our physical integrity. For instance, the blink that stops the spark of red hot metal hitting our eye as we stupidly grind a rusty lump of metal without eye protection, or it is the thing instinctively shifts our head to one side as we crash through an overgrown path with tips of branches coming at us at eye level. What goes down as instinct is our limbic system taking care of us, and it does this because it has been prepared since birth as part of our emotional system of basic trust to align our inner world and our environment. It is like the goldilocks and three bears sense insofar as it tells baby when things are just right not too hot, not too cold or when things are just right. The limbic system does this through the subtle interaction of different parts of our primitive brain. It activates hormonal flows that cascade through our bodies that prepare us for either for optimal awareness, dramatic life saving action, or sleep. These actions can be as subtle but necessary as the blink of an eye so we miss that spark, or the extension of our step so we don't slip on a wet path, or getting us to run pell mell from a herd of heifers that are frisking across a field at us, or to quicken or embolden our pace through a threatening city street, or playing dead when that bear approaches (Fig. 3.1).

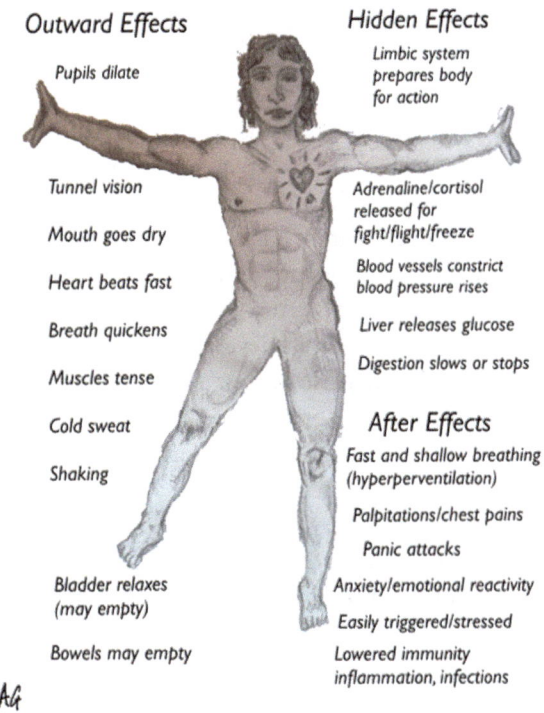

Outward Effects

Pupils dilate

Tunnel vision

Mouth goes dry

Heart beats fast

Breath quickens

Muscles tense

Cold sweat

Shaking

Bladder relaxes
(may empty)

Bowels may empty

Hidden Effects

Limbic system
prepares body
for action

Adrenaline/cortisol
released for
fight/flight/freeze

Blood vessels constrict
blood pressure rises

Liver releases glucose

Digestion slows or stops

After Effects

Fast and shallow breathing
(hyperperventilation)

Palpitations/chest pains

Panic attacks

Anxiety/emotional reactivity

Easily triggered/stressed

Lowered immunity
inflammation, infections

AG

Fig. 3.1 Fight, flight, freeze

Key Point—Proprioception

Proprioception provides our sense of where our bodies are in space. For example, that the chair is behind us as we sit down; that the next step is beneath our foot; that the door handle meets our hand; that our hand finds the light switch in the dark; like we can touch the tip of our nose or our ear with our index finger.

The Biology of the Limbic System

Let's see how the limbic system does its work in more detail, this will help us to understand how it responds to trauma and how we may work with its effects in ways that are creative and restore the balance that the limbic system was originally set up to hold on our behalf.

As will be seen in the diagram of the brain below, the limbic system is formed of some key components that nestle in the very center of the brain at the top of the brain stem, in what has been described as the reptilian brain, that part of us that developed early in our evolution that we shared in common with all creatures. The parts of this reptilian brain that make up the basics of our protective, fight and flight nucleus are the hypothalamus, amygdala, hippocampus, and the cingulate gyrus. What is deeply true about trauma and the brain is that *brain and body are one* and that body and brain are deeply and fluidly connected with each other. What needs to be held in mind here as we look at the brain is that it is just a part of this picture that encompasses brain, body, and our environment (Fig. 3.2).

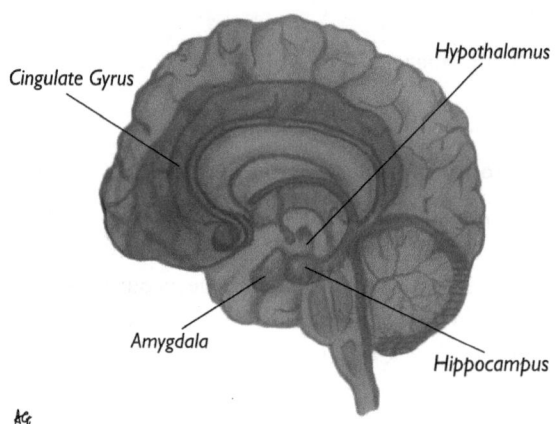

Fig. 3.2 The limbic brain

What Our Body Can Teach Us

If we pay attention, our body can teach us a lot about how to respond healthily to the stresses that follow trauma. Because body and brain are so interlinked traumatic events kick off a conjoined mental and physical response and after the extreme event our brain continues to instruct the body to kick into high alert when we are triggered by cues that remind us of the trauma. Knowing this we can actually reverse that process, we can consciously tell our body to tell our brain to relax and let go. Let us now look at each component of the limbic system in turn and what we can learn from them.

Amygdala

This almond-shaped organ sits above the hippocampus at the top of the brain stem and its tail loops around beneath the cingulate gyrus to which it is richly joined. The amygdala regulates our response to danger by kicking off a powerful physical response through the release of adrenaline. Adrenaline propels our fight-flight response, we leap out of danger before thought arrives, even before our visual cortex has registered what is coming our way, it is the very center that alerts and arouses us to action.

The other thing the amygdala does is to make us do things—to run away from danger and abandon the vulnerable, to tell lies to get out of impossible situations, and when we recall these things they can make us feel deeply ashamed. It is really important to allow a survivor to know that those shameful memories were not them in the best of times, it was them under extreme threat and it was the amygdala that made them run and enabled them to survive (Rothschild 2010).

When a threat appears the amygdala narrows our vision to just what is coming at us; like our ancient ancestors out hunting on the steppes, when a beast lowers its horns and charges we do not need to see the wide horizon, we need to narrow our focus to see exactly where to place the spear; or if in ancient forest when the mammoth turns to fight, we need to see the mammoth, not the trees. Our survival depends on focus, and these qualities of intense attention and focus have survived in us since ancient times.

How to work with this? The important thing to realize in this work with a survivor is that the amygdala triggers our fear response by releasing adrenaline. This is very intense but because adrenaline is a very short-lived hormone, it creates a powerful unstoppable response but its effects can be moderated and calmed through slow deep breathing, by reminding the person in the grip of it that they are *here* in the *present*, and if we give them something physical to hang onto—this can be a ring on their finger, a pebble in their pocket or some other talisman, it is possible to get to the other side of the dramatic re-living of past experience and to land in the present feeling safe and contained.

Hypothalamus

Lying at the apex of the primitive brain is the hypothalamus. The hypothalamus primes key organs such as the pituitary gland and regulates the ebb and flow of vital hormones through our body. It regulates our circadian rhythm, our inner time clock, that raises us in the morning, controls our level of alertness, and allows a slowing down toward sleep to occur in the evening. It controls appetite and hunger and regulates our temperature. It controls our thirst, causes us to sweat, and regulates how our kidneys absorb and secrete fluids. It sparks the release of stress hormones such as cortisol when we are under stress, and releases the key hormone oxytocin that stimulates trust and bonding. When we are in acute danger after the initial kick of adrenaline released by the action of the amygdala the hypothalamus boosts and maintains this through stimulating the adrenal glands to release cortisol. If you look at the diagram of the body "Fight or Flight" it can be seen how many of the fight and flight responses are regulated by the hypothalamus.

Learning Point

The Hypothalamus-Pituitary-Adrenal (H-P-A) Axis

The Hypothalamus-Pituitary-Adrenal (HPA) Axis orchestrates the flow of hormones that are key to our survival under threat and key to our recovery after stress. Under threat or stress the HPA axis is like the accelerator or gas pedal pushed down to the floor in a car, adrenaline is release that makes us hyper alert, and primed for action. If danger persists the HPPA axis stimulates the release of cortisol that keeps us on high alert.

High alert triggers the *sympathetic nervous system*, our fight flight response: blood pressure goes up feeding blood into our muscles; glucose is released from our body's stores, to feed brain and muscles; our lungs open, we breath rapidly powering the brain and muscles with oxygen; eyesight and hearing sharpen, focus narrows to the threat; digestion stops, we may empty our bladder and bowls involuntarily.

When the threat recedes the HPA axis triggers the *parasympathetic nervous system*, the body lapses into relaxation, blood pressure lowers, breathing slows, digestion resumes.

Hippocampus

The hippocampus has a bulb-like shape and sits right above the brain stem, where the spinal cord enters the brain, and curves in twin loops from around the interior of the mid-brain. Apparently its name is derived from the Latin for sea horse because their shape is similar. The hippocampus is the seat of our learning, memory, and spatial navigation. Like a telephone exchange it manages and co-ordinates key connections between memory and emotion within the cerebral cortex, the "thinking part" of our brain. Of profound importance is the role it plays in directing, anticipating, and creating imagined futures. From this position we can perhaps understand how it plays a role in trauma, laying down memories of shocking events and anticipating how to respond to both real and imagined threats.

Learning Point—The Plastic Brain

It is the hippocampus that is renowned as having a much greater volume among black cab taxi drivers who have to learn 'the knowledge' a map of London to qualify for the job. This fact also illustrates how plastic much of the brain is, and how it is capable of developing and rewiring throughout our lives in response to learning and environment.

The hippocampus is renowned for its plasticity, the way that it continues to develop, form new connections, and grow through life. Studies have shown London taxi drivers who must learn "the knowledge," a faultless working memory of the streets of London, have a hippocampus that is considerably larger than usual—in other words, the hippocampus grows according to need. At a very basic level it locates us in the world through the creation of spatial and emotional awareness and memory, it helps us follow directions, and it does this by integrating our senses and our reasoning capacities. It does all this consciously, but it is also constantly at work below the threshold of our consciousness, monitoring our sense of being in the world.

In the topsy-turvy world of trauma the hippocampus can pull current experience and memory so tightly together that a survivor can feel almost mad as if something that happened in that space over there and back then is happening right now. Gunshots on a country walk can throw a survivor into an utter panic. What happens is that memory and current experience become so bound together that they are as one with each other. It is this that can give someone in traumatic re-experiencing an overwhelmed and "locked-in" feeling as they focus on traumatic events.

How to work with this? Practice on yourself and then when the need arises if you are a helper or a therapist in the therapeutic moment invite the survivor to do this. Help them to stop and pause and open up their vision, to focus externally outside themselves, to look intently at you or something in the room, or something outside through the window. Invite them to take hold of an object, this can be the ring on their finger, some jewelry, a pebble in their pocket, or some other talisman that can help them to take their focus to the object and into the present. These strategies can help the survivor to break out of the locked-in attentional focus that traumatic re-experiencing causes.

As their attention widens they will de-escalate and relax. By doing this in a safe space, with a trusted person, in a repeated way a survivor begins to learn physically and mentally to let go of the traumatic triggers and the deep sting of associated memories. Follow this through, focus with the survivor and make deliberate sense of that was then, and this is now.

How to work with this Practice being in the now—this may be a moment outside when an intrusive memory erupts, or at home when a bad dream wakes a survivor up. It needs determination and courage to unravel these for a survivor who is caught up in what can be a terrifying re-experiencing of trauma but if we as therapist or helper are calm, and practical and warm, and offer careful and sustained empathic enquiry a new emotional experience can begin to emerge. Practice saying this: "That was now, we are here now, come back into this now." When they are alone or afraid to sleep or woken from a nightmare invite them to practice coming into the present, and invite them to keep a talisman or loved object close at hand to grab hold of and anchor them back into the present whenever fear erupts.

Cingulate Gyrus

Lying above the hippocampus is the Cingulate Gyrus that provides our autonomic or automatic functions, all the parts of us that keep on working automatically but need to be monitored and regulated such as the size of our pupils, and our breathing, blood pressure, digestion, urination, and sexual arousal. Most importantly it has a critical executive role in the quality of our thinking and our capacity for attention and plays a key role in motivation. It "decides" what is important to give attention to at any given moment of time, which is incredibly important when we are in danger and under threat.

So the cingulate gyrus plays a hugely important role keeping us alive without us even knowing it, sharpens our focus and narrows our thinking onto what really counts and after trauma whenever a threat lurks, imagined or real, the cingulate gyrus flares into action. This can be very unsettling for ourselves and those who live with us: our attention narrows so we miss the bigger picture; we leap into action when a threat looms. My wife is unsettled at how I almost always startle up from the chair when she comes into the house unexpectedly through the kitchen door.

How to work with this? Practice on yourself and then when the need arises if you are a helper or a therapist in the therapeutic moment invite the survivor to do this. Bring the startling thought or recollection into your mind and then breath into it. Very consciously open and expand the breath into your chest and widen your attention so you can hear all the sounds in the room, see all the qualities of light at play, feel the different textures and pressures that your physical body is in contact with. Rub your hands together and feel the temperature of your hands, massage your face gently and bring your attention there and look at whoever is there with you. This connection is so important because one of the things that we learn under threat is to avoid eye contact. This is something therapists and family members can watch out for—do we lock eyes when we meet, or do we glance, as if warily, out of the corner of our eyes before turning our full attention and meeting the gaze of the other? The shy glance can indicate trauma, possibly developmental trauma, it can also have cultural attributes, in some cultures children are taught not to look directly into the faces of adults or those of higher social status. However, good therapy will encourage us to step into the space with each other with open hearts and open faces and to gently enquire what it is that shuts us down from doing so. It will invite us to open up carefully, to feel into it, and enquire through felt sense what lies beneath. By doing this we can feel into what the cingulate gyrus is doing to us, notice it closing our attention, notice our blood pressure going up and our focus narrowing. Through gently but persistently noticing we can encourage the body to have a new emotional experience, it begins to learn or re-learn equanimity, to develop an inner eye on our body's unique self-regulation—and this can become homework, the survivor can practice as they settle, just noticing their levels of arousal and regulation in everyday situations, learning to be alert but equable.

Key Point—Through noticing we can encourage the body to have a new emotional experience, it begins to learn or re-learn equanimity, it develops an inner eye on its own regulation.

The Low Road and the High Road

Each of these areas of brain and body work together, the amygdala lying deep within the brain stem supplying the spark as it were, and then that spark orchestrated by the hippocampus, hypothalamus, and cingulate gyrus fluorescing through the rest of the brain, and carried through the body via the vagus nerve. In *Mindsight* (2011) Daniel Siegel refers to the low road and the high road of emotions: the low road being the unthinking emotional responses that erupt from the brainstem and the amygdala, the explosive and self-protective responses that include lashing out with irritation, anger, and rage, as compared with the more reflective high road of responses where the amygdala's response has been refracted by the hippocampus and cingulate gyrus into the thinking areas of the brain, which leads to a more reasoned, reflective responses where the intense emotions of fear, anger, irritation are modified by memory and thought.

Guidance

Breathing

Breathing slows things down, it lowers panic, and allows clear calm thinking to emerge. It is wonderful how it does this, almost magic but it's not magic, it is simple physiology, simple psychology, letting the body lead you to its calm place.

Breathing slowly and deeply sends signals to the cingulate gyrus that all is well, it tells the amygdala to stop being alarmed, and both tell the hypothalamus to return us to a state of calm balance, which tells the hippocampus to send waves of signals to the rest of the brain that ordinary thinking can return.

How to do it: sit with your feet firmly planted on the floor, your back held straight, shoulders relaxed. Alternatively, lie on the floor. Place your hands on your lower belly and breathe in, not a shallow breath into the top of your chest, but a deep long slow breath taken down into your belly as it were, so you feel your hands rising as the breath comes in, and falling as you slowly exhale. Count the breath in "One" and out "two". See if you can extend the out-breath so it feels as if you are breathing out long and slow. Keep counting and just follow the breath and the counting. If your mind flies off, stop and come back to the breath and begin counting again. See if you can get to "twenty" without your mind drifting off.

Learning Point

The High Road and the Low Road

Daniel Seigal named the instantaneous overwhelming self-protecting response of fear and anger as the **low road**, the thinking brain as the **high road.**

The **low road** is the emotional road that our amygdala triggers us onto without a moments thought when danger threatens either in the outside world or in our inner world. It happens without thought, and when fear is triggered our focus narrows, our attention becomes pin-pointed, we look only for danger.

The **high road** is the thinking part of our brain that kicks in when danger recedes. Instead of our reactions being governed by the primitive brain stem connections wash out into our higher brain. Our attention widens, a greater range of emotions flourishes, problem solving happens, new thoughts arrive.

After a bomb attack in his city that had injured him and from which he had narrowly escaped death Douglas felt incredibly angry much of the time. He erupted at his partner Zara and children with hardly a flicker of thought when they pressed upon him making demands or being too noisy. He couldn't bear this new eruptive, transgressive angry inner self and his family was often afraid of him. We did slow breathing exercises together—the whole family taking part, closing their eyes, Douglas breathed into the irritation and anger he felt; his partner and children breathed into their fear and alarm. After a week's breathing exercises at home supported by his partner he was really beginning to be able to slow things up: he could begin to see the buds of anger arising in him when he was triggered in a session: this was the amygdala setting off its alarms, setting of the adrenal system, flooding him with noradrenaline and arousing physical symptoms, tightness in the chest, stomach churning, his arms feeling full explosive of energy, and his mind beginning to cloud with anger. We stopped it there and brought Douglas back to the here and now. After quite a number of tries he really got it and he began to be really able to bring thinking to his experience. This was the "high road" kicking in, the hippocampus and the cingulate gyrus sending messages out into the rest of the brain where thought and reflection could begin to play a part.

Simultaneously, Zara and children were participating in the breathing exercises. For them the task was to be able to sit with his irritation and anger, and to see through their responses to his fear and his anger to a more reflective compassionate place. This sounds straightforward but it's not easy: fear and anger contend with each other, both are responses that protect us as individuals and in a family system, indeed in any emotional system (Flaskas and Pocock 2009), fear and anger can ricochet between people and amplify the felt experience, and mirror neurones play an important part in these emotional events.

Mirror Neurones

One of the powerful neurobiological systems at work in us is our mirror neurones. Located in the region of the brain responsible for movement these neurones function to anticipate the fulfillment of actions. For instance, if someone else lifts a glass to their lips the same neural pathways will light up in the brain of an observer. If you throw a ball for a dog and anticipate its trajectory the same neural pathways will light up in the brain of your dog. In humans this astonishing feat translates into the emotional sphere. For instance, if someone begins to cry the same neural pathways will light up in empathic people. It is thought that these qualities enable imitation, indeed they are powerful pathways for imitation; as such they enable learning imprinting patterns between generations from parents to their children, imprinting skills, social behaviors, and pathways of feeling.

In Douglas's family when he feels angry the motor-action part of his brain lights up and the motor-action parts of his family's brains light up too. In Douglas's brain fear triggers his amygdala, and the flood of adrenaline that stirs him into action he translates quite unconsciously into a readiness to fight and an overwhelming self-protective anger. It is overwhelming because it has taken the low road and he can't think. It is overwhelming because he is flooded with adrenaline and needs to act at lightening speed to protect himself. It is out of control because the effect of adrenaline within the limbic system is entirely selfish, it is about protecting oneself as a biological organism. The the will to survive as an individual kicks in and nothing else matters in that moment—there is nothing regulating Douglas's fear, he has no emotional connection with others, he has no connection with his social self, and he has no access to all the layers of his social learning. He is alone with his fear and his need to act to protect himself is paramount in those long seconds before the high road—the thinking brain—kicks in, and his family are right to be afraid. As the acting part of his brain lights up so do their's like this: fear, amygdala, limbic system. These are like billiard balls ricocheting around a snooker table. The point of breathing into these sensations is that the layers within the emotional system of trauma begin to reveal themselves and space for reflection emerges.

How Trauma Narrows Attention and Breathing Opens It Up

Under the influence of an activated limbic system our attention narrows to our own biological survival. However, when we breathe slowly and deeply into our abdomen this re-regulates our parasympathetic nervous system. When we breathe slowly and deeply deep into our tummy our heart rate slows, our blood pressure goes down, our digestive system begins to work again, our muscles relax, our attention opens up to everything around us, including those close to us. As we breathe into each of the sensations of fear and anger we see them for what they are, they are in fact just that, sensations to which through imitation and subtle learning we have attributed emotions such as fear anger anxiety. This isn't meant to downplay the reality, the impact, and meaning and value of emotions—it is simply that the breathing in opens them up to examination and allows us take a reflexive looking-in stance. In that reflexive, looking in space Douglas and the family became curious rather than afraid: in the slowed up space of the safety of the therapy session, each watched as Douglas's anger ricocheted into them and sparked off fear. We talked about it, and Douglas was able to see that his anger sparked out of fear—but that this happened at such lightening speed within him that he could hardly catch it: across the ether of the room and through the membraneous filter of his family's joint nervous systems, as they spoke about it, he was able to see it moving more slowly, how fear turned to anger—and that is when it began to stop.

We shall continue to consider more methods for slowing down this quick process of the amygdala. The thing with the amygdala is that it fires up in an instant. It's like stepping on a snake, the amygdala fires up the limbic system before thought gets anywhere close to starting up. You'd have to have eyes as keen and fast as a hawk to get ahead—but we can't see an ant crawling on the flagpole of the White House or a fly on the hands of Big Ben like they can. So we need to slow things down with breathing, and also things we will look at in later chapters such as bilateral stimulation, and keen therapeutic attention.

Douglas and Zara had a good secure base before the bomb attack, and our therapeutic work relied upon the family having an historical felt sense of it. Furthermore, Douglas had come out of a family with a secure base, and he and Zara had reproduced this, with the unique color of their own relationship, so when we explored Douglas's anger there was a sense that we did this knowing there was a secure base that could play with the ricocheting shocks of his misfiring amygdala. Finally, as he was practicing to do things better in therapy it was my role as therapist to play the parental part of being bigger, stronger wiser, and kind—and to delight in their exploration.

The Vagus Nerve

Almost the final thing to mention in this chapter is the vagus nerve. This is the nerve that runs down through the body from the brain, carrying messages to the throat, heart and lungs, skin, and digestive system. It keeps everything going in the background but after trauma it is very activated by the hormones released by the limbic system. It triggered but deeply background activity helps to explain why after trauma survivors suffer from stomach upsets, panic attacks, palpitations, tightened throat, loose bowels, and skin complaints. These are all hidden signs of trauma.

Learning Point

The Vagus Nerve

The vagus (wandering or vagabond) nerve is the main nerve fiber highway for the parasympathetic nervous system. It proceeds out of the brainstem and wanders down through the body via the larynx (throat and voice box) heart, lungs, stomach, intestines, bladder, and skin, where it controls our sweat glands. It is part of the autonomic (automatic) nervous system that regulates heart, breathing, body temperature, and other vital organs.

It explains why after trauma and under chronic stress we may suffer from many complaints linked to the actions of an over alerted vagus nerve: constricted throat; palpitations; rapid shallow breathing;

---

nervous tummy and guts; loose and irritated or constipated bowels; skin complaints.

Body Work

For therapists, because the limbic system and vagus nerve are completely over activated in most survivors it is deeply important to work with the body, notice bodily symptoms, enquire into the sensations they feel, soothe, and show how to soothe. Use psycho-education to make the link between traumatic events and bodily signs and symptoms. Teach relaxation and breathing, and suggest the survivor does body work as an adjunct to psychotherapy—this can be massage, yoga, reflexology, and other things to which they would be open. In addition prescribe running, swimming, or walking everyday, as early in the day as possible.

What We Can Do as Family and Friends

Consider all this together with the survivor and in your family/friendship circle, take turns to speak, listen, and reflect.

Understand how basic trust may be broken after trauma.
Understand how the reptilian brain acts to keeps us all safe.
Consider fight, flight, freeze—how does that play out with you, what are you fight, flight, freeze moments. Consider this together taking turns.
Pay gentle attention to what alarms and triggers.
Can we notice what narrows our attention and what opens it out?
Practice narrowing, focusing, and practice opening out.
Can we be warmly engaged but not in charge of the process?

Notice how fear and anxiety come in waves—stay with the survivor as they ride out the waves, let them come to a place of calm through breathing; practice breathing together, it's good for everyone.

Breathe into your abdomen, breathe in for **seven** and breathe more slowly out for **eleven.**

When the low road kicks in, practice the high road: invite someone to be your low road/high road guide and mentor, and you be their's.

Practice how to soothe yourself, and be soothing.

Be kind to the vagus nerve, relax, breathe, gentle touch, massage.

Ease away palpitations, tummy troubles, with breath work, relaxation, massage.

Go running, swimming, practice yoga, stretching, massage: do it all this together.

References

Crittenden, Pat. 2008. *Raising Parents: Attachment, Parenting and Child Safety.* Cullompton, Devon: Willan.

Flaskas, Carmel, and David Pocock. 2009. *Systems and Psychoanalysis.* London: Karnac.

Rothschild, Babette. 2010. *8 Keys to Safe Trauma Recovery.* London: Norton.

Schore, Allan, Daniel Seigel, and Louis Cozolino. 2021. *Interpersonal Neurobiology and Clinical Practice.* London: Norton.

Sroufe, Alan. 1996. *Emotional Development: The Organization of Emotional Life in the Early Years.* Cambridge: Cambridge University Press.

4

Creating a Welcome

As we have seen in the first two chapters when anyone has been traumatized the sense of disconnect from others can be huge; there's almost a double sense in this, first a feeling that one is massively distanced from the safe secure self that one used to be, where life was safe and predictable, and secondly this undoing of our safe self is often wrapped up in the additional sense that what has happened to us is one of a kind, so completely singular with all its vivid features that it can't be imagined, understood, or appreciated by anyone who hasn't been through it. Feelings of shame and helplessness can add to this sense of alienation, of an unbridgeable gulf between self and others. The same feelings can affect families too, making it hard for them to put things into words between themselves, creating distance because each family member will have had their own unique experience of the extreme events that have affected them all. Finding the common ground in a shared traumatic experience can be hard when some in the family feel shame for not being safe or protective under severe stress, or for leading the family into danger. In addition, when a family member is alone in having had a traumatic experience the sense of this feeling of being alone with the experience can be

J. Woodcock, *Families and Individuals Living with Trauma*,
Palgrave Texts in Counselling and Psychotherapy,
https://doi.org/10.1007/978-3-030-79039-4_4

exaggerated by the sense of aloneness they felt at the time of the trauma, as we considered in chapters one and two, that psychological sense of abandonment when one's protective internal parent evaporates in the middle of an extreme event.

For all of these reasons it is hugely important to make a traumatized individual or family welcome. It really needs to emphasizing for therapists who are schooled in ways of therapy that promote a setting where the therapist takes a detached observing and overtly neutral stance that this should be set aside in favor of creating a warm welcome, to emphasize through words and gestures and attitude that the individual and family have "landed on a rock," an utterly trustworthy place, where their experiences can be heard, understood, and weighed without a rush to judgment.

Guidance

Creating a Welcome

You are welcome	Listen without judgment
Reach out, go the extra mile	Pay attention to felt sense
Be a warm and emotionally connected therapist or helper	Do your best to understand
	Move at their pace, be led by them, take time

This is equally true for a family's response to a traumatized family member. Set prejudices and judgments aside based on your familiar stories, rooted in what you know so deeply about each other and open yourself up to listen in a warm and engaged way to what their *new* experience has been.

It is really important for therapists, or helpers, and family members to understand that when someone has been traumatized they may be unlikely to respond to offers of help in a straightforward way, their basic trust may have been shattered, and because of this they may be unlikely to respond easily to the usual overtures of trust. They may appear to be flaky, unreliable, ambivalent, and untrustworthy, they will almost certainly need you to reach out to them. When family members reach out to someone in the family who has been traumatized be warm and concerned, and don't be surprised by rejection and ambivalence—stay warm, play the long game. As a therapist don't be surprised if they fail to show up to your formal appointment invitation. You may have to go the extra mile—reach out, telephone, show warmth, and concern.

Learning Point—It Is Hard Listening to Trauma

It is hard listening to trauma, especially when it's someone we love; hearing the risks they ran; their closeness to death; their ways of coping that may seem strange and bizarre; hard to hear the shame they may feel. It is triggering for us, we have to work hard to keep an open heart and mind.

One woman who had been serially raped in detention took seven years to settle into therapy and to work directly with the trauma, she came at first with her partner, and then with her young children. We worked elliptically with the effects of trauma on their relationships, and only when she was really settled and re-qualified and back in her original profession did she call back to say, "Now I really want to work with what happened to me." Similarly, men in a platoon that had been decimated in Afghanistan took as long as ten years to really begin to engage in psychological work, and through the intervening years their families, friends, and comrades stayed in touch and kept on linking them to help, and kept on hoping.

However, while reaching out with warmth make sure that simultaneously you hold onto the curious observing questioning self. Therapists consider attachments in the family, how do they enter and greet you, do they fill the room or hold back, who opens up and takes the lead, who is retiring, how much consideration does each one shows for other family members sensibilities? We know from attachment studies that the moments of arrival and departure project the shadows of individual and family attachment styles and the questions to be asking are:

- What is their attachment style?
- Has their attachment style been altered by extreme experience?

We will consider attachment in even greater depth in chapters that follow.

Containment and Validation

When we are focused on scary sensations and emotions we need containment and validation. Containment is the sense and knowledge that the person helping us is able to see with their mind's eye, and feel in their guts, and understand with wisdom what we have been through. It is a deep attunement to our emotional experience and an empathic response to the range of our feeling. It is also the capacity of the therapist or helper to bear the pain of what is being said, and to emotionally digest our experience. Containment also conveys an unconscious appreciation that the person helping us is like an ideal parent, bigger, stronger, wiser, and kind. Validation is the other element, it is the developing gut knowledge that this person will believe us, that they will gently but determinedly explore our experience, and open doors into aspects of it that we might have thought closed because to think about it was unbearable.

Learning Point

Containment and Validation

Containment—an attuned emotional response to our feelings, the capacity to bear the pain of what is being said, and to emotionally digest our experience.

Validation—when the shape of our experience is seen and understood in the mind and in the heart.

Containment and validation are therefore two poles of a therapeutic experience that is so important in work with trauma; only with good emotional containment can we open up and find that our experience is validated, and in validation we discover a deeper experience of containment. For instance, a young woman had her throat cut by a gangster who wanted to terrify her mother into submission. The young woman couldn't believe how her mother had exposed her to such terror, and she felt deeply ashamed by what had befallen them and by the life they led. Slowly she began to appreciate that the therapist while being deeply compassionate was making no judgment about all the imperatives of their survival. He saw them for what they were but his focus was on emotional understanding, not moral judgment. The young woman realized this at a gut level and felt contained. As a result, she was able to say more about their life and to get hold of the ambiguity of her experience in a way that validated her experience and was forgiving and redemptive of both herself and her mother.

Bordered Experience and the Exiled Self

What this example throws up is how often trauma hits people living at the margins of society, where experience outstrips social norms and this can lead to a struggle to have one's experience validated. This is so often the case with trauma: social norms are very powerful and easily exclude those who do not appear to fit in. Consider Vanessa a homeless woman in her late thirties, she had two daughters who felt proud of her but they also felt deeply concerned about her vulnerable condition. She had given them a stable upbringing but then things went badly wrong, the sexual abuse she had endured as a child came crowding back in on her, she lost her job as a community worker and then her flat. Her ebullient personality enabled her to survive on the streets almost buoyantly for several years but homelessness took its toll. She said, "I was pigeonholed as a homeless person, people rarely saw through to the whole of me as a mother, former community worker and a person with a host of life experience. I was a puzzle, even to myself and it was only in consciously making the connection to my abuse through counselling provided by a homelessness organisation that I began to recover real mental equilibrium for the first time in my life." Vanessa had exiled the abused part of herself for many years in order to survive, she had partitioned it off in an unthought part of herself but its troubling energy had shown itself in feelings of shame, low moods, slightly manic episodes, and bad dreams. Her counselor offered her the containment and validation that allowed her to retrieve the exiled unthought and unfelt parts of herself. It was painful to work uncovering and making the connections between her abuse and her fluctuating moods but when she eventually shared it with her daughters they understood deeply and instinctively. They experienced Vanessa as being able to bear the pain she had previously avoided and having strengthened her capacity to contain and validate her own experience in a way they found deeply moving and affirming.

Gaze Aversion

Gaze aversion is the term Louis Blom-Cooper used to describe the host of helping agencies that failed to notice that four-year-old Jasmine Beckford was being systematically starved and beaten to death by her stepfather and neglected by her mother. It is a good term that sums up what happens to us when we fail to see something clearly because it is too shocking and painful, and doesn't fit with our preconceived beliefs. Gaze aversion is a way of dealing with cognitive dissonance when a situation is so shockingly out of kilter with how we believe things should be. It is a way of categorizing experience in a way that excludes the stuff that doesn't fit with or beliefs, as in the case of Vanessa. It is also the experience of many people of color who find that the range and depth of their life experience is left out of the reckoning. Take Anselm who was raised by his beloved grandparents in Jamaica and when he was six without warning or preparation was sent to the United Kingdom to join his father and mother who had not seen him since he was six months old. He ran screaming from his mother at the airport and had to be caught as he dodged through crowds of people in the arrivals hall. His parents were dismayed by what they deemed as his disrespectful behavior and they never bonded. He spent years pining for his grandparents who he never saw again and his withdrawn and downcast demeanor was read by his parents as poor conduct and he was frequently chastised and later beaten. What was a terrible case of disrupted attachment grew into a childhood of emotional misunderstanding, alienation, and despair, which hardened into serious emotional neglect. Later it was a gang that gave Anslem a sense of belonging and identity and his anger was such that he was an easy conduit for violence and a terrible series of traumas flowed from that. He was angry that he was only seen as a big black dangerous young man and his many woundings and slights, and his frustrated love and loyalty and tenderness were never seen. Furthermore, the richness of his very mixed life experience was ignored and he was seen as he described it, "Like a one dimensional man."

Another quite different example of this sort of phenomena was the soldiers who returned to Britain from imprisonment in the Far East after the second world war, who found that while there was general sympathy for them there was very little realistic appreciation of the appalling suffering they had been through, it was as if it couldn't really be conceived and in the celebration of peace the rest of the country just wanted to move on. American soldiers returning from Vietnam experienced something similar with the added complexity that people were horrified by events in Vietnam and public sympathy for the war was exhausted.

Frequently work with trauma requires us to engage our imagination to encompass the exiled selves and bordered experience. This can be applied directly to refugees who find that the variety and depth of their life is literally left on the other side of the world because of the cultural norms that do not allow them to bring the fullness of their life into exile.

With all these examples there are two sides to what is going on— one side is exclusion because of gaze aversion, discrimination, racism, failure of empathy, lack of imagination, and impoverished social justice. Another side is the way that exclusion and shame work together to rob us of the confidence to be really present in our lives and to live them out in their fullness. These matters make it so important that we offer a welcome in therapy and counseling where the fullness of experience and personhood can be encountered, and as we have seen this is a matter of attachment, neuroscience, cultural norms—held in mind to offer a welcome that provides containment and validation of all life experience.

There is good evidence that even families with optimal attachment styles prior to trauma will find those altered by extreme events. Sheila

Melzak (1999) describes one young child who said of her father, "He looks like my dad, smells like my dad, has my dad's voice but he's not like my dad anymore." Similarly, Elise van Ee (2013) measured the effects of trauma on the attachment styles of refugee mothers and fathers, and saw that in many cases their emotional bonds with their children were stressed by extreme events. In particular, parents were discovered to be on a continuum where the quality of parent–child interaction tried from disconnected parenting where parents were dissociated and that parents who showed more overt symptoms of trauma were less sensitive and structuring [containing] and more hostile to their children. However, we need to hold in mind that also many parents respond to trauma with a great deal of resilience but what these observations bear out is the need to pay sensitive attention to attachment styles, and to hold in mind that signs of hostile or withdrawn attachment may well be affects of trauma, and that if one "reaches through these" with commitment, and warmth a better outcome may emerge where there is a deeper attainment between everyone involved because of the trust that is developed.

What We Can Do as Family and Friends

Consider all this together with the survivor and in your family/friendship circle, take turns to speak, listen, and reflect

Ask how are we welcoming, can we do things differently?

Ask in the circle, how can we welcome this crisis into our lives, what can it teach us, is it an invitation to do things differently?

In the face of a crisis are we likely to do the same, but try harder at it, or can we do things differently? If we do things differently who will have their foot on the accelerator and who on the brake? Can we see that both are necessary and valuable?

Listen without judgment, as far as you can

Practice being emotionally containing as you can; invite someone to be your emotionally attuned, responsive mentor, be theirs too

Remember its hard to listen to trauma, be kind to yourself

Discuss in the circle what experiences are easy to look at and validate, and what's harder and how come?

References

Melzak, Sheila. 1999. The Emotional Experience of Violence on Children. In *Violence in Children and Adolescents*, ed. Ved Varma, 2–21. London: Jesica Kingsley Publishers.

van Ee, Elise. 2013. A New Generation: How Refugee Trauma Affects Parenting and Child Development. Utecht University Repository. http://dspace.library.uu.nl/handle/1874/284735.

5

Trauma, Attachment and Resilience

In this chapter we draw out the similarities and differences between developmental trauma and event-driven trauma. Developmental trauma is extreme events, sometimes one-offs but most commonly continuous situations of danger and neglect that occur in childhood that shape our inner world and contribute to who we are, our sense of identity, and the very filters through which we experience the world. By contrast event driven traumas are extreme events that happen to us outside of the course of our expected development, often in later life. These extreme events may profoundly change us and, as the chapter will explain, often in ways that are very similar to developmental traumas. Developmental trauma has a lot to teach us about event-driven trauma, and the work that has evolved to resolve event-driven traumas can teach us a lot how to work with developmental traumas. We will start with an appreciation of developmental trauma as it has been understood from within attachment theory.

© The Author(s), under exclusive license to Springer Nature
Switzerland AG 2022
J. Woodcock, *Families and Individuals Living with Trauma*,
Palgrave Texts in Counselling and Psychotherapy,
https://doi.org/10.1007/978-3-030-79039-4_5

Attachment

The key ideas that underpin recent thinking about developmental trauma have emerged from attachment theory that has been based on research into how early relationships with our caregivers shape our attachment styles. The thinking goes that if we have optimal relational experiences with our caregivers we will develop an attachment style that is characterized by being free and autonomous. What this means is that we relate to people with openness and with a sense of freedom to our emotional experience and to theirs. This means that we more easily attune to other people's inner worlds and more easily let them into ours but in so doing they can't capture us, we feel able to come and go and deepen or loosen our commitments in a way that feels emotionally balanced and true to our intentions and equally respectful of those with whom we form relationships. Research over many years suggests that our attachment behavior settles into a clear style by about the age of four, and that this style remains consistent over the course of our lives in all our meaningful and intimate relationships.

Learning Point

Optimal Attachment

Child is autonomous and free, and engages freely and easily in imaginative play	Mother and child are adaptable
Child is free to go to and fro from the mother and explores readily	Mother and child's shared strategy is to maintain emotional contact with each other
Parent recalls memories easily and describes her emotional life in an open and coherent way	Mother and child are emotionally comfortable
Both mother and child show their true feelings and know their true feelings

---

> Feelings and thoughts are
> experienced coherently

Avoidant Attachment

We can also be raised with less optimal attachment styles and these variations most likely occur because our parents have their own less than optimal attachment style. Two distinctively different styles have been noted by researchers one is described as avoidant or dismissive, the other as ambivalent or preoccupied. In the avoidant style it is noticeable that parents are experienced by their children as a bit scary, and typically when reuniting after a separation it is noticeable that a child that has developed an avoidant attachment style will be wary of its parent, catching sight of them out of the corner of their eye, rather than with a full on welcoming gaze; they will also be careful about how they approach in conversation and play, automatically checking out in micro-seconds if the parent is in a safe and approachable mood; other key features of this attachment style is that the child has somehow learned that emotional closeness can be risky and so an attachment dance develops close but not too close—a key to understanding this is to see the child as having developed a strategy for keeping themselves safe while maintaining a relationship with their parent that meets their basic needs.

This avoidant attachment style will follow us into adulthood; we will find ourselves almost unknowingly being cautious about how we engage in friendships and intimate relationships, watching from the edges rather than diving in, checking out we're liked, being alert to other's mood, feeling rejection all too easily.

Learning Point

Avoidant Attachment

The person with an avoidant attachment is likely to have forgotten much of their childhood but confusingly for the uninformed observer they will actually tend to idealize it. However, this idealization of their childhood does not fit the actual care they had as a child. For instance, a mother is described as wonderful, but when they were a child a boy could not tell his mother of any serious harm that happened to him because his mother would have been angry. In the avoidant attachment the child's attachment behaviors are deactivated, it unconsciously learns to be pseudo-independent and rejecting, and it avoids closeness, and in adulthood there is denial of past pain. As an adult they are dismissive of emotional closeness, rejecting of emotional approaches, and emotionally distant with a disengaged transactional style. The shared strategy of parent and child is to avoid emotional or physical closeness and the child is reserved, avoidant and compulsive in behavior. There is a mismatch with memories intact but feelings about those memories may be distorted. Furthermore, the avoidant/dismissive parent may appear detached to an observer but they are experienced by the child as too close unless distance is kept.

Ambivalent Attachment

The Ambivalent attachment style is the last we will consider for the moment—this is typical of the child who is raised by a parent whose emotional availability is uncertain. As a result the child learns to win their attention, and to hook the parent in so their needs are met. The result is a child who is insecure about whether it is loved; although the parent may be outwardly committed to parenting they often drift off into preoccupied states of mind and lose sight of their child's needs, or they are distracted by other pressing needs and put their child second. It doesn't matter if this happens occasionally but when this is the overall manner of the parents style the result is a child that has to work hard to be parented and in later life someone who becomes a partner who is insecure about being loved and may enact all sorts of subtle strategies to keep their loved ones hooked in and interested.

Learning Point

Ambivalent Attachment

The main characteristic of an ambivalent attachment is a preoccupied and entangled parent. Although the parent is committed to parenting they are often emotionally unavailable. An observer may think parent and child are close, but the parent is most often actually experienced by their child as emotionally unavailable which provokes clinging. The child learns that the parent will respond but only if they work at it. The child's strategy is to keep close and force the parent to notice them by being demanding and/or overly babyish. The parent is characteristically preoccupied, often ruminating on unresolved issues from the past. Parent and child monitor and "mind-read" each other in an attempt to forestall the other drifting away. Threats of pushing away or abandonment are very effective short-term strategies to reinforce closeness because they activate attachment behavior. This push/pull threatens the security of the child. The price of mind-reading, push/pull, and threats of abandonment is a loss of autonomy for the child. In summary, the child's attachment behavior is over activated; the parent is preoccupied and entangled in the past, and the parent has an incoherent sense of themselves and of their stories of the past, and they are only intermittently available. This sets up a child who is reactive, passively resistant to emotional overtures and at worst coercive. Furthermore, the outcome of ambivalent attachment is one's true feelings are hidden and distorted.

We need to be cautious about over describing these forms of attachment—they tell a lot about us but they are not the last word about who we are. They are underlying psychological tendencies that shape us in relationships but they do not capture the complexity of who we are. Furthermore, we have to bear in mind that positive relational experiences through the rest of life can profoundly influence our attachment style. This could be a redeeming relationship where an older adult such as a teacher or mentor has taken an interest in us and clearly given us an experience of being held in mind; it can be a romantic relationship where we experience love and care with someone who is robust enough to withstand the emotional push and pulls of our attachment style, and it can be counselling or psychotherapy that enables us to become more reflective of how we are in relationship. In all of these scenarios the key attribute that can cause a shift in an attachment style is the opportunity for insight to be brought into an old pattern of behavior out of which a new emotional experience can emerge. For example, David Quinton and Michael Rutter (1988) compared how the prospects of young men who have been in care with multiple disrupted attachments were transformed over the long term when they were in relationships with well-adjusted young women as compared to young men who didn't have such secure romantic relationships whose outcomes were much less good. In another example, Egeland (1988) describes how an emotionally containing relationship with a senior such as a teacher, youth leader, or mentor, where one is simply held in mind can transform a troubled young person's prospects. The need for something best described as ordinary human kindness is so important here, and not as a one-off but the kindness that persists, so the young person has an enduring sense of being held in mind in a positive, loving, and uplifting manner.

Key Point

The avoidant child has a certainly unavailable parent, whereas the ambivalent child faces an uncertainly available parent.

John Byng-Hall Child Psychiatrist and Psychotherapist (1995, p. 117).

Attachment and Trauma

Understanding attachment sets the scene for understanding the under-lying dynamics of developmental trauma and event-driven trauma. Two very positive and encouraging themes that can be pulled out of our understanding of ordinary secure attachments are of deep importance here. The first is the way in secure attachments infants and their care-givers each hold the other in mind in a positive way. There is a sense in which for both baby and mother the other exists in a lively, responsive way in their mind when they are apart and this sets the scene for when they are reunited. There is an expectation when they meet of mutual pleasure, reciprocal responsiveness, and acceptance. There is also a sense of a shared emotional narrative, in simple terms that mother and baby love each other in an uncomplicated way that can be put into actions (smiling and looking at each other with pleasure, and being responsive) and words. This contrasts with a less securely attached mother and child where in an ambivalent attachment the child may need to hook in a mothers attention, and where despite her ongoing lack of responsiveness a mother might quite rightly claim she always loved her child and where feelings of abandonment are pushed beneath the threshold of conscious-ness for child and mother so there is a less coherent emotional narrative. It also contrasts with the avoidantly attached mother and child where the child actively avoids attention because attention can mean either emotional or physical harm. In that scenario researchers have noted the negative feelings both experience about each other are denied, and this too leads to an incoherent emotional narrative.

Learning Point

Being held in mind

| The other is recalled with pleasure | Being at an event or place may bring them to mind |

There is accurate recollection of their qualities	They are bought to mind in a physical way, thoughts of them may infuse the heart, the chest, the tummy with feeling
There is an accurate sense of the relationship	

Developmental Trauma and Event-Driven Trauma

As the name suggests developmental trauma is the bad things that happen to us as we grow up that leave their mark and can profoundly shape our way through life. Developmental traumas include emotional neglect, physical and sexual abuse, family violence, and domestic abuse. In these situations the child quite unconsciously develops a way of being attached to their parent while keeping themselves safe. This is most likely to be the situation of the insecurely attached child who experiences their parent as unsafe and scary and even actually dangerous. As we have seen above for the ambivalently attached child the danger is mostly one of emotional neglect, of being overlooked because their parent is preoccupied, but this can also show itself as physical neglect as well when a parent is out of touch with what a child needs to be physically healthy. For instance, a distressed and depressed and preoccupied parent who isn't regularly making nutritious meals.

In comparison, event-driven trauma can be described as traumatic events that happen to us outside of the usual run of life such as accidents, natural disasters, warfare, human rights violations, and other life threatening and near death experiences.

Learning Point

Resilience in the face of adversity: the factors that protect us against the lasting effects of trauma

The ability to integrate experiences into our belief systems	Interaction with others in securing gains
The presence of self-esteem	Parental modeling or modelling by other supportive adults
The ability to be proactive in relation to ongoing stress	The ability to process events and experiences in a meaningful way
Having secure affectional relationships	Gaining mastery over stressful events is itself a powerful form of resilience
Some measure of success and achievement	

Resilience to Trauma

The key factor that stands out in all traumas that determines whether it lodges in children and young people in a way that deeply affects them is whether there are adults around them who can protect them from its worse effects. If adults can make sense of it for children it becomes understood and intelligible and most importantly if they have the emotional wisdom that can help them to process its emotional effects. Adults and importantly parents who model calm, thoughtful resolve in the face of adversity pass that calm resolve onto the children around them. These ideas about how adults model resilience for children are important for families caught upon disasters described in Chapter [x].

As Michael Rutter has explained in his paper *Resilience in the face of adversity* (1985) protective factors are deeply important and can make us psychologically resilient in the face of trauma. When we consider the list of protective factors we see that all of them will be provided in a family with optimal attachments, whether they will all be provided in families with ambivalent or avoidant attachment styles is far less certain. However, children may also be good at winning support from others or they may be fortunate to have other adults in their life who offer them aspects of resilience.

For instance, John's parents were deeply neglectful of him but his aunt and uncle took him away on holiday every year, where they played family games that they clearly enjoyed, they went on long walks, he learned to cycle with them, they took an interest in his learning and education and bought him books and read him stories, they talked about his interests and participated in them, enjoying what he would do. They were like an island of light in his life; with them he was esteemed, he was secure in their affection for him, they talked to him about life and he could problem-solve situations with them, and he saw them doing all of these things with each other. This was the redeeming relationship that allowed John to move forward in life and later to make a good and deeply affectionate relationship with his partner. At a physiological-neurological level, in the ways discussed in Chapter 3, John's uncle and aunt made good use of their mirror neurones to attune to him emotionally; their calm well-regulated inner life that washed with adrenaline when there was genuine fun and excitement, gently sparked off the parasympathetic nervous system, and then easily reabsorbed the adrenaline and cortisol through the sympathetic nervous system as play and excitement came to an end and they headed for calm, rest, and relaxation. It could be said that with his aunt and uncle John experienced his amygdala, hypothalamus, hippocampus, cingulate gyrus and vagus nerve working together in a well-orchestrated way, the amygdala keeping him alert when he was excited and at play; the hypothalamus regulating his HPA axis in an optimal way, washing him with the ebb and flow of excitatory and alerting hormones, and bringing him back to rest; the hippocampus stimulated by play, and conversation that linked all the events in his life together; the cingulate gyrus quietly at work in the background keeping his breathing, heartbeat, and digestion in synchrony; his vagus nerve doing its thing linking head, heart, and guts. Thanks to his aunt and uncle John grew up with a well-modulated gut instinct, and an open heart that made sense of the world, and all the stories that came his way.

The Circle of Security

The other thing at work between John and his uncle and aunt was a fundamental attachment process that is at work in all family settings, which is the *circle of security* that is beautifully described by Bert Powell and his colleagues (2016). It works like this, at best parents (and carers and other adults) provide a secure base for their child. The child sets out from that secure base to explore the world. As they do this they need their parents to support their exploration, to watch over them, delight in them, help and enjoy them as they play and explore. At some point the wandering, exploring, playing child begins to feel uneasy and needs to head home to their secure base. At this moment the parent needs to welcome their child back, to protect, comfort, and delight in them, and most importantly help the child to organize its feelings.

In this whole process it is important that the parents are bigger, stronger, wiser, and kind; that whenever possible they follow their child's need, and whenever necessary they take charge. It also bears repeating that two emotional ingredients already stated are really important, which is the parents need to *delight* in their child and parents need to enjoy *with* them. If these processes are in place a child knows it is loved and appreciated, that it has a secure base. This secure base isn't merely something a developing child appreciates it is the bedrock of a good relationship between a couple, and the fundamental basis of good family life.

Learning Point

The circle of security

- The child sets out to explore from (the parents/carers) their secure base

- The parents support their exploration, they watch over, help and delight in and enjoy *with* their child

- The wandering child feels uneasy and needs to head home to their secure base

- The parent welcomes them home, protects, comforts and delights in them and helps the child organize its feelings

Resolving Childhood Abuse in Adulthood

Things don't always go well though, but in the recovery from childhood neglect and trauma we can be helped by the ideas that run through the whole of this book. Andrea was neglected as a child, along with her three brothers, and they stuck together like a gang, but she was singled out by a neighbor who befriended her it seemed, although what happened when she was twelve was that the adult male in the household began to sexually abuse her until she was fourteen and managed to get away. Breaking through the shame and silence terrified into her, she managed to speak to one of her brothers who was sufficiently persistent to reach through the emotional wall she had put around herself. Nothing happened to the abuser, and Andrea wasn't helped at the time, she and her brothers just didn't have the support and self-belief to push for help, neglect had confused and silenced them. In her early thirties struggling again and again in intimate personal and sexual relationships Andrea eventually talked to a friend and this led, a year or so later, to her picking up with a therapist. The therapist understood three things, that Andrea's childhood neglect, which Andrea actually dismissed as being serious, resulted in her having only a slim narrative grasp of her childhood experiences, what this meant was that the stories of her life were thin, truncated, and often confused. This was largely because there had been no emotional and intellectual-cognitive coherence in the emotional system her parents had provided, and this had been amplified by the abuse she suffered, and the scrapes she got into later, things didn't hang together easily in Andrea's life. The second was that Andrea's limbic system was on full alert, and she was skillfully watchful, so one might have hardly noticed the third thing, which was the character of her attachment style was anxious and dismissive, but this showed itself as the work deepened in the way she was poorly attuned to her own emotional currents, and rather dismissive of what her therapist might have described as the emotional truth of intimate situations: she preferred to play, to bat things away, to keep intimacy at a distance, rather than fully landing and opening up. This beautiful, intelligent, sensitive woman was like a frightened bird, armed with an electric fast cat's, scorpion claw. The fourth aspect about

Andrea was that she lapsed into dissociated states, and sometimes had panic attacks.

Guidance

Resolving Abuse in an Adult Survivor

Value dissociation as a safe place	Using relaxation and calm as places of grounding
Finding other safe places in one's mind	Working with the window of tolerance
Finding safe objects that ground one in the here and now	Paying attention to the flow of intimacy between therapist and survivor
Coming and going from these safe places	Working relationally, keeping the clunk out of technique; technique as knowledge that flows
When the abuse comes to mind being able to move in and out of a safe place in the mind, and so to emotionally re-regulate	Creating coherent narratives out of disjointed experiences and stories of growing up
Paying attention to the ebb and flow of the limbic system	Paying attention to emotion and staying emotionally connected

---

The therapist was deeply acquainted with the work of Yvonne Dolan, described in *Resolving Sexual Abuse* (1991) which is solution-focused and deeply Ericksonian hypnosis informed way of working. In many ways this thinking is a precursor to the newly emergent work based in neuro-biology and the physiology of attachment and the limbic system. It was within sexual relationships that Andrea dissociated, going somewhere safe in her mind, away from the bodily memory that sexual intimacy called up. She was safe but she realized as she fell in love that this wasn't a satisfying form of intimacy for her partner, she was somewhere else, and when called back to real intimacy, she was upset and disturbed. The therapist had her value this escape but over months of work, they breathed into these spaces to bring her into the present in a way that was safe and emotionally contained, while the therapist at first, using their gut instinct, and then with Andrea together they mapped out how her limbic system kicked off, created dissociation, which was like another room in her mind, where she was safe and detached, and then brought her back into a new emotionally safe, properly validated and safe present. They invented safe places together, coming and going from them, while the therapist payed accurately attuned attention to Andrea's state of arousal. This had a twofold benefit, firstly the therapist modeled an attuned parental figure, secondly the therapist charted the ebb and flow of Andrea's limbic system, bringing her into an appreciation of a well-regulated emotional experience, where she felt the therapist intimately in touch with her inner world. This was deep relational work, that was never clunky or technique led. Although the technique was deeply there, it flowed into the therapeutic conversations, and these conversations did another amazing thing, they charted a narrative for Andrea's inner world and her experience in relationship that had a connecting rationality that fitted into the narrative of Andrea's attachments in ways that are similar to the ways charted by Rudi Dallos and Arlene Vetere in *Systemic Therapy and Attachment Narratives* (2009). As they recognize what is joined up is the feeling space, the limbic system, our ways of attaching and detaching, and disjointed narratives of family life are faced, worked through, and made more coherent.

If we go back to Chapter 4 although the issue wasn't sexual abuse but war trauma we can see some parallels of this work with Douglas and Zara. However, instead of working with the historical situation as in Andrea's case, with Douglas and Zara the therapist was able to work with the live situation with the family, as Douglas's limbic suit rocked out of control and he dissociated into a place of anger, where he lost connection with their emotional reality in his mind and that repelled his family into limbically fearful places. The therapist offered the therapeutic space as a place of safety, this included their frank acknowledgment of his aggression and anger and the fear it induced in his family. It was a therapeutic relationship that stayed connected to emotional reality, while modeling understanding and acceptance that had limits, Zara and the children in conversation with Douglas were the monitors of what was acceptable.

The family breathed its way in and out of its places of safety, calming Douglas's overactive amygdala and the way this ricocheted around the family as an emotional system, and out of this work, and the work of recollection a more coherent experience was fashioned.

What We Can Do as Family and Friends

Consider all this together with the survivor and in your family/friendship circle, take turns to speak, listen, and reflect

Practice holding family, friends, and survivor in mind. Reflect, how does that feel, in my head, in my throat, in my shoulders, in my heart, in my breathing, in my guts, and in my legs and feet?

Be a circle of security, allow exploration, welcome each other in, enjoy together

Create a safe place, ask how do we make this safe?

Take opposing views, take turns to play the devil's advocate, shake the differences out, gently

Learn and teach relaxation; invite someone to be your relaxation guide and mentor, and you be their's

Listen without judgment and an open heart, emotional attune and validate experience

Notice and celebrate all the things that make you resilient

Learn, as my friend the psychotherapist Jane Cutler says to "focus on the numb places, there's a lot of intelligence in there." Do this gently, with calm and compassion.

Stay connected, watch the things that pull you apart, breath into them, and let them go

References

Byng-Hall, John. 1995. *Re-writing Family Scripts*. London: Guilford Press.

Dolan, Yvonne. 1991. *Resolving Sexual Abuse: Solution-Focused Therapy and Ericksonian Hypnosis for Adult Survivors*. New York: Norton.

Egeland, Byron, Deborah Jacobvitz, and Alan L. Sroufe. 1988. Breaking the Cycle of Abuse. *Child Development* 59: 1080–1088.

Powell, Bert, Glen Cooper, Kent Hoffman, and Bob Cooper. 2016. *The Circle of Security Intervention: Enhancing Attachment in Early Parent-Child Relationships*. London: Guilford Press.

Quinton, David, and Michael Rutter. 1988. *Parenting Breakdown: The Making and Breaking of Inter-generational Links*. Beatty, Nevada: Avebury Books.

Rutter, Michael. 1985. Resilience in the Face of Adversity. *The British Journal of Psychiatry* 147: 598–611.

6

When Secure Attachments Are Blown Apart

In this chapter we plot our way through what happens when otherwise secure attachments are blown apart by traumatic experience. The stage is set for this with a summary of some more key thinking from attachment theory. We begin with the notion of coherence, which we have understood in previous chapters has a twofold property. On the one hand in its most straightforward way it merely shows how a story that hangs together in a way that makes sense, and here is meant the stories of our lives, the narratives we carry in our heads that shape our ways of being in the world, of how we filter and order experience (Dallos and Vetere 2009). In other ways it is about how implied by that word filter coherence is a deeper experience of the emotional sense that is made of things, often below the threshold of language and consciousness because these experiences were deeply part of us before we could bring language to them.

J. Woodcock, *Families and Individuals Living with Trauma*,
Palgrave Texts in Counselling and Psychotherapy,
https://doi.org/10.1007/978-3-030-79039-4_6

Coherence

The attachment researcher Mary Main (1991) noticed that something she described as coherence is really important in the development of a secure attachment. Coherence is the ability to understand the world of relationships in a way where everything fits together in a reasonable and understandable way. Furthermore that coherence comes from not only things being explained clearly but by there being a fit between the way relationships are explained and the way they are lived. Also that the inevitable puzzles and difficulties of relationships are explained in ways that are open and friendly rather than in complicated, hidden, and hostile ways. At best coherence describes a warm family atmosphere in which stories about family life are shared freely, openly, and with fun and humor. Coherence also means that there is an emotional fit between the moods and ups and downs of family life and how they are understood. Even more deeply, it implies that a parent has a coherent story about their own upbringing, asking them to bring a key moment in their life to mind such as a question from the adult attachment interview like, "Can you remember what would happen when you were hurt physically?" And you would expect them to be able to recall an incident and clearly describe how their parents responded to care for them. As part of this looking back one might expect the child to be able to see pretty clearly into the desires, motivations, and emotional responses of their parents.

Metacognition

A key to being able to experience coherence is the child's capacity to be metacognitive. What this means is our ability to look in on our own cognitive (thinking) and emotional (feeling) processes. Another word for it would be the ability to be reflective, to look in on our own states of mind. This first of all requires that we can tolerate our own states of mind, that we aren't so angry or frightened or overwhelmed and upset that we can't look in. Sometimes we will be overwhelmed and it is either our own ability to acknowledge or begin to acknowledge how we feel or it may take others around us to provide an acknowledgment of how feeling and behaving that allows us to settle and look inside. Mary Main describes the process of gaining metacognition like this: before the age of three most children don't have the capacity to be metacognitive, and because they can't look into their own thinking and feelings this means that they can't deduce the feelings, thoughts, and motivations of their parents or caregivers. As a result events and emotional situations are experienced in very concrete ways. It is our capacity to step back from ourselves and look into our own inner experience that enables us to appreciate things from another perspective, like, "Oh, it could be like this, or it could be like that…" This metacognitive ability turned on our own processes of thinking and feeling enables us to deduce that other people share this same capacity to be reflective. Indeed Peter Fonagy (2002) in his research work on mentalization reckons that from a very early age babies and children learn to anticipate what is going to happen. To paraphrase it, "If I cry, she'll come, when I smile, she smiles back, if I winge she'll feed me" and so forth and in this way a predictable inner world develops in the reliably parented baby in which they have a sense of influence over the behavior of their carers. Fonagy describes the baby as having a developing capacity to think ahead—in very young babies this is hardly thinking in the mature sense of having well-formed concepts but the beginning of thinking, a bodily awareness of self and its influence on others, and as months and years pass this develops into thinking, especially when that proto-thinking is responded to in a warm, responsive, and reliable manner.

Learning Point

Metacognition and Mentalization

Metacognition—being able to stand in a different part of our minds and look in on our thinking and feeling, to think about our thoughts and see our cognitive (thinking) and emotional life as a process

Mentalization—being attentive to others so that we are able to "see and feel" into the minds of others; being able to determine their motives for actions and even anticipate their actions and responses; being able to fairly accurately guess at the emotions others feel

The process that develops is that as babies learn to predict and influence the world, they appreciate that in their little world they exist in the mind of another and another exists in their minds. This profound, early experience lives at the core of our early experience in a myriad of ways and is at the heart of metacognition.

Dual Coding

Another developmental layer that Mary Main describes is dual coding. At its simplest and most general dual coding can be described as the ability to "see" something in one's mind from more than one perspective. Things can have more than one quality. They can be present and absent; they can be aunty or mummy's sister, they can be good and bad. Mary Main suggests that prior to the age of three children cannot dual code. For instance, you may be familiar with the developmental psychologist Jean Piaget's experiments in object permanence, whereby a child cannot track a favorite toy hidden under a series of cups, when the cups are swapped around the child can't follow which cup it is hidden under. The same happens in relationships insofar as mummy or daddy seem to disappear when they leave the room. These moments turn on this failure to dual code: things are present in a very concrete way or not present at all: they cannot be imagined in the mind as having more than the present quality. Because young children cannot dual code they do not have the capacity to be metacognitive, that is they cannot "see" their own thinking. Similarly, to extend the idea, they cannot be meta-emotional either, that is, they cannot be truly reflective of their own emotional experience. In other words being metacognitive and meta-emotional are developmental achievements (Woodcock 2000).

Key Point—Dual Coding

The ability to "see" something in one's mind from more than one perspective

---

Developmental Trauma and Forgetting

It almost goes without saying, that if the adult is the source of suffering, if they are the one who is rejecting, violent, sexually abusive, or neglectful then the consequences for the child or young person can be very much worse. It is children who survive such circumstances that will tend to have stressed attachments and to exhibit attachment patterns described above as either insecure and avoidant. They in turn are at risk of passing these same attachment patterns onto their children. Furthermore, what attachment researchers have noticed is that when people with insecure attachments are questioned about their upbringing there is very often a denial that things were bad. This is not just a veneer of normality that is smeared over a challenging childhood but actually part of what it means to be insecurely attached. In insecure attachments because there is no coherence between what is being felt and experienced it is very hard for a child's emotional experience to be validated. For instance a violent or neglectful parent may be still a protector and provider, and connection to them provides security but at a high cost, and the conflicting feelings are not validated and are literally pushed underground, there's literally nowhere to go with the experience.

> **Key Point—Forgetting**
>
> We forget things or do not even install them reliably in our memory when the story of what happened is not clear and consistent and there isn't clarity and coherence between what we experience and what we feel, and when our feelings and experiences are not validated or brushed over or are even actively denied

The securely attached child has a parent who holds them in mind, who provides a coherent emotional account of family life, where there's a fit between events and how they are explained and understood. For the insecurely attached child none of those things are given. Furthermore, lack of coherence compromises a child's ability to dual code and develops reflective capacity, and where there are overwhelming extreme events dual coding is even more deeply compromised: things aren't simply forgotten or brushed under the carpet they just don't survive in consciousness. Naturally this comes at all sorts of different levels of intensity.

What Happens in Trauma

If we now apply these ideas to extreme events we see that in the same way that prior to about the age of three children cannot "dual code" and therefore they cannot be metacognitive in the moment of an intense extreme experience adults lose the capacity to be reflective and to dual code; our thinking capacity is literally overwhelmed; our ability to emotionally comprehend the enormity of the threat to ourselves and others is swamped; the instinctive, protective reptilian brain kicks in and bodily survival becomes the priority and all other considerations are subsumed by the pre-eminent need to survive. Of course there are shades of this, but for the most traumatized, this is the effect of an extreme event. In the midst of extreme events we lose the capacity to dual code the experience and hence our capacity to be metacognitive to the extreme events is compromised. Extreme events are therefore experienced, and recollected when they can be, in a very concrete way.

Learning Point

What happens in trauma—a summary of attachment

Bodily survival becomes paramount	Reptilian survival brain kicks in
Capacity to be metacognitive is lost	Basic trust—our belief in a fair and decent and safe enough world is lost
Capacity to dual code (to experience things from many perspectives) is lost	Our internal mother deserts us: no-one seems to be holding us in mind

---

Capacity to be reflective is lost	Our internal "attachment telephone exchange is bombed out'
Thinking is overwhelmed	Feelings of fear and anguish are overwhelming

So, after extreme events we lose our way developmentally and our previously intact capacities are damaged. This is true of the most securely attached and previously well-adjusted adults when the extreme event has been sufficient to overwhelm us. It is as if our innermost development core, our attachment nexus, our emotional telephone exchange has been bombed out. As my colleague Sheila Melzak a child psychotherapist described (1999), children might say of a mother who has been traumatized, "I know she's my mum, but she's not like my mum used to be," and this is because the power to reflect has been compromised, that space between a stimulus and a reaction has been telescoped together so the space in the mind feels overcrowded and overwhelmed by stimuli. When we lose the capacity to dual code because of trauma the events we have endured take on a very concrete quality, trauma is what it is, it has a particular valency and anyone else's right to challenge that experience no matter how trusted, be they partner, children, friends, or therapist can be experienced as deeply problematic. Furthermore, highly expressed emotions, alarm, fear, and other roused states easily overwhelm the survivor and their capacity to reflect and endure the ordinary demands of attachment without stress and irritation are easily lost.

Learning Point

Valency

In chemistry valency means the combining power of separate elements.

In trauma valency means the psychological bonds that an extreme event creates in the mind and body of a survivor. The loss of the ability to dual code means that those bonds are experienced in very concrete and almost pre-reflective ways.

For example, we hear a gun shot on a country walk and we lose our train of thought and begin to tremble: the sound brings a recollection that triggers a deep bodily response—memory and bodily response are bound together.

For example, the door crashes open and we are startled, our breath is taken away, we back away: the sound triggers a recollection and a bodily startle response and fear—bodily memory of crashing doors, and recollections and bodily reactions are bound together.

When Trauma Detaches Us

Alana was really badly beaten by people smugglers while she was crossing North Africa, she saw and endured terrible things that she would prefer not to talk about, including killings and people dying from neglect and abandonment. The boat across the Mediterranean foundered and people drowned, in particular a woman and child, who had become her friends: she was heartbroken by not being able to help them. Alana had enjoyed a really secure, good upbringing but politics and war in her homeland had forced her to flee. She was an architect's assistant, fairly newly qualified but also experienced working in a team putting up schools and clinics. She had a really good grasp of how teamwork between different professions made things work, and of bringing ideas alive by working with stakeholders in the community. But she was blown apart emotionally by her multiple experiences—the gratuitous violence she had seen and experienced was beyond anything life, even in her war-torn homeland, had prepared her for. In exile she had a couple of very brief relationships with young men but she just couldn't hold it together—she sought comfort but she was jumpy, suspicious, highly alerted, nervousness, and this is what finally bought her to therapy. She described how the sweet, strong young man she had been seeing finally said no because she just wasn't able to relate to him in a way that had the deeply connected intimacy she seemed to promise from more of a distance, and she described how something felt dead inside her. She knew her ex-partner was right—she just couldn't connect. She was jumpy, irritable, had nightmares, and could be sleepless but she was also sort of alright too, she could still get on with people but she was no longer any good at closeness, and she felt deeply alone. She'd get in touch with home by telephone but felt quite detached from her devoted mother and father, it was like they just didn't quite exist in her mind any more in quite the same way.

Alana was a bit of a mystery, to herself, on lots of levels she was really together, but on other levels she was completely in pieces, and this is often true in trauma. For the therapist, and for family and friends, it can be tempting to overplay the survivor identity to the detriment of the part of Alana that was suffering, and this is particularly so when like Alana survivors cope well in the external world of work and play but the most difficult aspects for them are the manner in which they relate differently after the trauma in intimate relationships. For Alana this showed itself with the young men who fell for her, and in her conversations with her family back home. These were aspects of her that weren't so easily apparent to those who were more distant from her, and it speaks to the need to attend to intimacy in the therapeutic relationship. Alana found this changed intimate part of herself puzzling and difficult to put into words. She could speak fairly easily of flashbacks and weird mental phenomena, of shocking dreams that startled her awake. We worked with those with methods we will describe in later chapters, but the attachment and trust issues described here show how our most intimate connections with ourselves and others can be blown apart by trauma. Let us try and understand.

As we have seen to be metacognitive means the ability to be able to look in on our own thinking, feelings, and experience as if from a second position outside ourselves, we might call it taking a birds-eye view, or simply being reflective. Because we are able to be metacognitive, we are able to *dual code*, which means to see things as having more than one property or meaning. Mummy's sister can also be my auntie, the dog can be friendly but can also bark very loudly, mummy can love me but also be cross sometimes. Dual coding means that the good and bad can co-exist in people and things, and of course this capacity to understand the co-existence of properties develops with more sophistication as we mature. The opposite of dual coding is when we experience the world in very concrete ways and we can't nuance the textures of experience and of relationships, for instance, people are seen as purely good, or bad. Dual coding underlies our ability to understand metaphors because metaphors represent a thing being something else, for instance describing heavy rain as "raining cats and dogs." Dual coding lies at the heart of play, for instance, the "peek a boo" game when we hide our face behind our hands that relies on the cusp of development where a child can't quite dual code, we are literally there or not there. Dual coding allows us to "flex" in relationships, to enter the dance, to move with the flow.

Learning Point

Metacognition, Dual Coding, Metaphor and Play

- Being metacognitive—being able to look in on our own thinking, as if from outside ourselves, might also be described as being reflective

- Dual coding—when things have more than one property that can co-exist together, for instance uncle is daddy's brother. The capacity to see things from more than one angle is the capacity to dual code

- Metaphor—when phrases and have another meaning. For instance, "looking daggers" is a hard, aggressive look

- Play—when we play we dual code, things take on multiple meanings, for instance a carton top is a boat, a rug on the floor is an island. Play is the beginning of metaphor

- When trauma is transformed into metaphor it begins to lose its capacity to hurt us

However, a deeply traumatic event can so easily compromise our ability to dual code. The events itself are experienced in various singular ways that seem all too concrete. In addition because of this "concrete effect" of the loss of dual coding we experience ourselves as totally alone with the experience: it is almost as if the loving parent who accompanied us through our growing up disappears: a rather dry description of this is that "our attachment nexus" is disturbed, or even temporarily destroyed. Our attachment nexus means the net of relations we have internalized that hold us together and provide templates for our relationships. These are deeply compromised and simultaneously because of the loss of the capacity to dual code we respond to events and relationships in very concrete ways. Because being close to others thrives on nuance and play, relating intimately becomes very hard work, especially when we feel so fundamentally alone. This is what had happened with Alana, this is why her parents felt so distant to her, and she felt so distant to them; this is why her relationships with boyfriends felt so clunky and difficult and unsatisfying—she just couldn't dual code, the playfulness had gone out of her, she felt devastatingly alone, and she constantly experienced the sensation that no one could attune to her experience. This complex experience is what the theories discussed in this chapter suggest was Alana's experience, and it truly fitted what emerged as we delved into her experience behind the raw fundamentals of anxiety, fear and flashbacks, all of which played their part in her suffering and recovery as well.

This has been a rather theoretical but important chapter. In the chapters that follow we will trace out the ways we can support our loved ones and loosen and untangle these deep valent over-connected bonds of trauma and help to put in place the scaffolding for recovery. We consider how other survivors like Alana emerged into full survivorhood in later chapters.

What We Can Do as Family and Friends

Consider all this together in your family/friendship circle, take turns to speak, listen, and reflect

Ask and discuss, how do we sit quietly with a strong heart and mind? Consider that you do not have to be passive in the face of this challenge. What are the positive things about stillness, and what are the positive things about activity? What stirs us to action? What stirs us to calm?

Take opposing views again, take turns to play the devil's advocate, shake the differences out, gently.

Be reflective, practice seeing the other point of view.

Practice standing in someone else shoes, and then back to your own.

Practice patience, breathe into it.

Help the survivor's story come together in a coherent way, gently.

Be understanding of a survivor with a bombed-out attachment telephone exchange.

Play, play games, set puzzles, draw, sing, be creative.

References

Dallos, Rudi, and Arlene Vetere. 2009. *Systemic Therapy and Attachment Narratives*. London: Routledge.

Fonagy, Peter, György Gergely, Elliot Juris, and Mary Target. 2002. *Affect Regulation, Mentalization, and the Development of the Self*. New York: Other Press.

Main, Mary. 1991. Metacognitive Knowledge, Metacognitive Monitoring, and Singular (Coherent) vs. Multiple (Incoherent) Model of Attachment: Findings and Directions for Future Research. In *Attachment Across the Life Cycle*, ed. Colin Murray-Parkes, Joan Stevenson-Hinde and Peter Harris. London: Routledge.

Melzak, Sheila. 1999. The Emotional Experience of Violence on Children. In *Violence in Children and Adolescents*, ed. Ved Varma, 2–21. London: Jesica Kingsley Publishers.

Woodcock, Jeremy. 2000. Refugee Children and Their Families: Theoretical and Clinical Approaches. In *Post Traumatic Stress Disorder in Children and Adolescents*, ed. Kedar Nath Dwivedi, 213–239. London: Jessica Kingsley.

7

Trauma, Pain, and Transformation

In this chapter, a model of thinking about traumatic vulnerability and pain is carefully thought about. The model is used as a guide to help survivor, family friends and therapist to map a way through from overwhelming symptoms such as panic attacks and flashbacks toward recovery.

When Georgia got home from a very challenging foreign assignment she found she was not sleeping well, she didn't want to meet up with friends and she fell irritable a lot of the time, not that she had even properly clocked the irritation, it was her mother who noticed it on a visit, and also commented on the fact that she was unusually withdrawn and preoccupied. This woke Georgia up to what was happening and she realized she had been captured by some events she had covered while working abroad as a journalist. One was of two children in a family she had got to know really well who had both been killed by shell fire. Georgia realized that the images and feelings of distress and loss she felt for the girls and their parents and surviving brother and sister were constantly playing through her, and another was of the constant grinding demoralizing effect of the war, the hopelessness and ever present

J. Woodcock, *Families and Individuals Living with Trauma*,
Palgrave Texts in Counselling and Psychotherapy,
https://doi.org/10.1007/978-3-030-79039-4_7

danger she had lived through: she realized she had a horrible gnawing pain deep inside and a slow thud of recollections passing though that hit her almost physically deep inside. Most tellingly and often accurately true after trauma was that she hadn't actually realized anything was really wrong until she and her mother had argued when her worried mother had probed and questioned a little too insistently. What Georgia realized was that she was in terrible pain, grief for those two little girls and their family, hopelessness of that war-torn country and the terrifying time she had spent there.

Pain Is Not Pathology

Babette Rothschild (2010) makes the very important point that pain is not pathology. What she means is that the psychic and emotional pain that we feel after trauma should not be regarded as disease or damage. In fact, pain is a most natural response to trauma. What we need to attend to with care is that the pain is not so overwhelming and that it can't be properly acknowledged.

Learning Point

Pain is not pathology but it can drive us into pathological ways of coping with it. Emotional pain lights up the same regions of the brain that fire up when we experience physical pain. We can turn to substances that deaden pain to help us manage the psychic pain of trauma

Alcohol

Drugs

If someone is over-using or misusing alcohol or prescription and non-prescription drugs this may be a way of trying to manage an earlier trauma.

Highly stressful events cause the anterior cingulate cortex that sits in the mid-brain to light up and physical pain lights it up too, and its rich connections with the limbic system and other brain areas reveal its role as a co-ordinator of bodily and emotional responses to stress and pain and trauma.

When we hurt ourselves unexpectedly, such as stubbing our toe, our reactions are most often instinctive and involuntary. We yell, we clench our toes, we hop about, and eventually, as we gain awareness we rub the injured spot. Furthermore, just as our toes contract in an instinctive and physical manner we also literally withdraw from the scene in our mind. We find it hard to return to the moment of impact, and we curse whatever it was that got in the way. Cursing actually helps.

Key Point

Our instinctive response to pain is to withdraw, contract our body, and hunch up.

We do almost exactly the same with emotional pain.

In this description of physical pain our involuntary response of withdrawal and contraction is very important to consider because we do almost exactly the same with emotional pain. As Jon Kabatt-Zinn (1990) one of the founders of Mindfulness who devised the mindfulness and pain relief program at the University of Massachusetts Medical Centre describes, our instinctive response to pain is to withdraw, contract our body, and hunch up. As we do this we create the conditions by which we lose the opportunity to learn from pain. Of course, once burned we learn instinctively not to go near the fire again or if we have stubbed our toe to walk with care when we go barefoot.

However, what Jon Kabat-Zinn shows us is that if we stay with the sensations we call pain and move beyond our instinct to withdraw and close up, we discover that there is a cascade of sensations, such as heat, throbbing, sharpness that follow. If we open up and just allow those sensations to come through into consciousness we discover that they become more diffuse. We in turn are no longer "in pain" in the sense of being consumed by it but we are now merely the observer of these sensations that we have so readily called pain. Now the pain is separate from us, it has become a set of sensations that are uncomfortable but open up more slowly to a different outcome than simply cursing blindly at our misfortune as we hop about with a banged toe, or shin, or thumb, or head.

We understand from pediatric medicine that very often liquid paracetamol is given to children who are in pain and discomfort, and very importantly for us to note, often the discomfort is more in the nature of emotional discomfort than frank physical pain. For instance, it is often given to children who are grizzly and sleepless. Parents may not be quite sure what is causing the child's restlessness but sure enough liquid paracetamol sends them happily off to sleep it seems. This is complicated, because by doing that the child is slightly sedated and often it may be not physical pain and discomfort that is being covered up by the drug but emotional discomfort. In this way, the family system learns subtly and unconsciously that painkillers mask emotional pain.

Guidance

Staying with Pain

If we stay with the sensations we call pain and move beyond our instinct to withdraw and close up we discover that there is a cascade of sensations, such as heat, throbbing, sharpness that follow.

If we open up and just allow those sensations to come through into consciousness we discover that they become more diffuse.

We in turn are no longer "in pain" in the sense of being consumed by it but we are now merely the observer of these sensations that we have so readily called pain.

Now the pain is separate from us.

Delve into the discomfort, see that as you enter it, rather than resisting it, that there's a lot going on, a skein of intertwining physical and emotional factors that get twisted up into a thing we call pain.

This is quite a long way from Kabat-Zinn's approach. What has happened is that we have disappeared down the complicated rabbit hole of pain—by contrast he would say something like this: delve into the discomfort, see that as you enter it, rather than resisting it, that there's a lot going on, a skein of intertwining physical and emotional factors that get twisted up into a thing we call pain. He's not suggesting that we endure pain with gritted teeth, or never dose our children or ourselves with pain killers—he's merely inviting us to pause and mindfully delve into the sensations and emotions (and by the way, as we learned in earlier chapters emotions are sensations) and that this mindful approach can lead us to a place where all the skeins untwist, and we find ourselves bearing pain and discomfort in a more open-minded way.

This thinking is equally true of emotional pain, taking pain killers actually does help with emotional pain, as do anti-depressants and along-side these approaches delving in mindfully also helps too. For years doctors have noticed how patients with depression often come to them with back pain, abdominal pain, and other painful physical ailments. These pains are very real but they are also physical manifestations of depression, anxiety, and other matters that have emotional origins, which can also emerge from traumatic origins. So let us take this journey of pain slowly and see how we can learn about traumatic events and pain.

Being Safe

We also need to be cautious with these insights because something else that is really important is that we need to be safe enough to work through trauma. After returning from her assignment abroad, Georgia felt phys-ically safe for the first time in many years. Nevertheless, when she was debriefed she felt very upset as she described the worst of what shad happened. However she passed off those feelings as temporary and threw herself into preparing to go abroad again but something stopped her every time an assignment was passed her way. It was at this moment that she argued with her mother and her pain and discomfort flooded into consciousness.

Georgia was now ready to feel and think and talk about what had been troubling her but getting to this critical moment had been neither obvious nor easy. We can lay out some of the conditions that had brought her to this point and the factors that her family, friends, and loved ones needed to consider to support her through to the point of opening up and working through the trauma and beyond.

We need to be safe in order to open up and face our physical and emotional pain. We also need to feel safe in order for the traumatic material to surface in a way that makes sense. Making sense means that we experience the things that we think, and feel and do as being linked in a way that has a rationality. When we are traumatically unsafe, the things that we feel and do are somehow not linked. We react in ways that feel out of control or in ways we cannot quite fathom. Reactions surface in us that seem odd and uncanny. Sometimes our odd and out of the ordinary responses may be more obvious to our family, and friends, and loved ones, than to ourselves, as was the case with Georgia.

Key Point

When we are traumatically unsafe the things that we feel and do are somehow not linked. We react in ways that feel out of control or in ways we cannot quite fathom. Reactions surface in us that seem odd and uncanny.

The Need for a Secure Base to Work Through Trauma

Being safe demands a few simple requirements, yet for some of us they may not be easy to achieve. According to the American psychologist Abraham Maslow, our need for safety is fundamental to our sense of self. He knew all about this because his own family had fled the Tsarist persecution of Jews in Russia at the turn of the twentieth century and as a boy in New York he had to contend with anti-semitic gangs. It could be said that this compelled him to work out a psychological system that would explain the conditions we all need not only to survive but to thrive (Fig. 7.1).

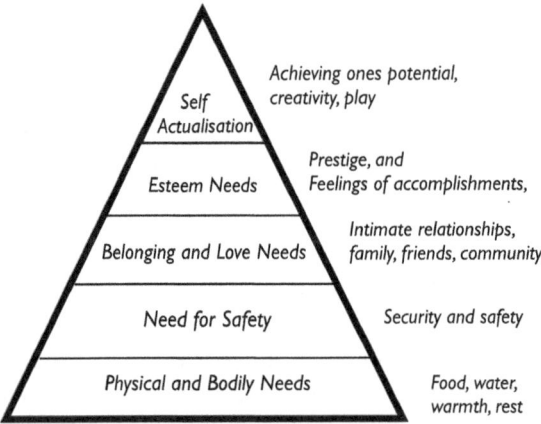

Fig. 7.1 Maslow's hierarchy of needs

Maslow reckoned that when our basic needs are met we are then in a position to thrive and to self-actualize. What he meant by self-actualize is the capacity to grow into ourselves and reach our potential. His thinking fits with traumatic experience very persuasively. Only when our basic physiological needs such as food, water warmth, and rest are met can we move on to establish security and safety, and only when those needs are met can we open up to establish and maintain our needs for belonging such as friendships, intimacy, and other reciprocal relationships. Finally, only when belonging is in place can we move toward higher needs and goals, what Maslow described as our need for esteem, accomplishment, and ultimately creative self-actualization in which we achieve our potential.

Holding Maslow's model in mind can enable us to have a nuanced conversation with Georgia about her readiness to work with her trauma. What aspects of her basic needs and needs for safety required attention and strengthening before the work could go ahead? The key here, as always, is that Georgia needs to be in charge of the pace and direction of this healing work, and able to meet the challenges it would throw up at a pace that worked for her. The other very important point is that all these needs are not only real and objective needs they are also symbolic needs. For instance, some of us might feel quite safe living in a tumbledown hut in the woods, but some of us need a solid property around us. Some of us might feel safe living in a neighborhood with gang warfare going on, some of us want leafy suburbs. Some of us may like a solitary life, others of us want to feel our friends and family are close at hand. Rather oddly trauma can move us in two directions, either toward wanting more security or toward neglecting our safety and seeking out danger.

Meeting Physiological Needs

Meeting the survivors' physiological needs is the starting place for work with trauma. Not until the base of the triangle is in place can we move up.

Panic Attacks

Returning to Georgia's we can see that her physiological needs were met at a basic level, but she suffered from panic attacks that undermined her sense of physical security. Objectively she was safe: symbolically she was in danger all the time.

> Objectively Georgia was safe: symbolically she was in danger all the time.

Panic attacks occur when we are triggered by obvious external cues that remind us of trauma or more subtle internal cues such as a memory or a resemblance that has an association with the trauma. This kicks off the limbic system that primes us to respond in fight/flight mode. However, because the danger is symbolic and held in the memory, there is nothing to fight or flee from, so our body escalates its response into panic that seemingly comes from nowhere, and this is deeply unsettling and upsetting. It is as if the body has a life of its own independent of our control. The effects are so dramatic that some people feel as if they are going mad. This can be intensified because the panic attack can trigger flashbacks and fugue states where partial memories and physiological reactions like tastes, and smells, and sensations of the trauma flood in.

Guidance

Panic Attacks

The trigger can be a sensation, memory, that connects to the trauma
Physiological effects—rapid shallow breathing; dizziness, rapid heart beat, intense fear.
  Remedies
1. Immediate remedy—concentrate on breathing making it slow and even; breathing into a paper bag watching it inflate can help; breathe in slowly through the nose for seven seconds, hold the breath for several seconds and then breathe out slowly in an extended way through the mouth for eleven seconds. Keep doing this until calm arrives.
2. Remind yourself this is a panic attack; you are not in danger; you can take back control by breathing.
3. Longer term remedy—take a brisk walk or run of at least half an hour first thing in the morning, and in the late afternoon if you can. This burns up accumulated stress hormones that can trigger us. It re-regulates our breathing, heart-rate, and relaxes our general physiology.
  Once we have used the immediate remedy to overcome a panic attack they become much easier to manage and we may be able to more easily spot when our breathing becomes shallow panting and dys-regulated and to go for a walk and/or do some breathing exercises to bring it under control.

At a simple physiological level what happens in a panic attack is that we begin to over-breathe, with rapid shallow breathing that saturates our bloodstream with carbon-dioxide. We feel dizzy, our heart rate shoots up, and we may believe we are having a heart attack, and fear that we are going to die, we may also have an out of the body experience. These sensations are powerful and dramatic but they can be managed.

Meeting Safety and Security Needs

Once Georgia's panic attacks began to stop and felt less dramatic they lost their grip on her and she began to feel she had achieved a good degree of physiological security. However, there were still things that made her fearful. She didn't like to sleep in a house alone and did her utmost to avoid it; she also slept with her room door open so she could listen out for danger; she wouldn't venture anywhere after dark unless she was accompanied. These needs were so powerful that they felt like compulsions.

Following Maslow, we can see that these immediate "felt" dangers Georgia experienced had to be a prominent aspect of the early work she did. She needed to be released from these compulsions that made her life so complicated to organize. For instance, if her city flatmates were away she would travel back to her parents to stay. She felt conflicted and infantilized by these requirements.

Visualization, Breath-work and Relaxation

Visualization, breathing and relaxation are beautifully simple ways of enabling a survival to establish a sense safety in the mind and body. Georgia was invited to bring up the triggers that were alarming her, made her feel safe enough in my presence to visualize them and then we used breathing and relaxation to enable her to let them go. She took the procedure home with her and practiced between sessions, deepening her capacity to relax and let go. Sometimes this is enough, sometimes more intense procedures like EMDR described below are indicated if the memories of the trauma are triggering, or avoidance of traumatic cues is interfering with life or emotional numbing is part of the everyday picture of life.

Exercise

Visualization, Breath-Work and Relaxation

1. Invitation to imagine a safe place making it as real as possible in ones mind, feeling it in ones mind and body, embodying it; entering it and leaving it. Being empowered to come and go from that place of safety.
2. Establish a relaxation method
3. Visualize the traumatic triggers, the things that make one feel unsafe. Feel them, embody them, re-experience the key aspects of the trauma.
4. Breath into the visualized trauma—moving toward a place of relaxation. Use the safe place if a sense of panic or overwhelm threatens.
5. Work forwards and backwards through cycles of this work until all the panicking triggers are quelled.
6. Imagine oneself alone with the traumatic triggers able to move backwards and forwards into a relaxed mental space where one feels confident.
7. Use breath-work and relaxation, let everything go and move into a relaxed and safe mental space.

Flashbacks

The next step in establishing Georgia's sense of objective and symbolic safety was to tackle her flashbacks. She hadn't admitted these to her mother or friends because they often felt slight, almost like deja vu although occasionally they had been powerful and strong. Flashbacks are sometimes vivid, like a film unspooling with sound, smell, and sensation that completely obliterates the present moment. But more commonly they cover a whole host of uncanny physiological sensations, startle responses, memories and blended partial memories, and sensations. They can leave the survivor feeling maddened, almost insane because they are so unpredictable, or they can be uncanny fears that intrude in specific circumstances, like the feeling of apprehension that may overtake us when walking in a wood as dusk approaches.

Whatever their character flashbacks can be described as the past visiting in a way that is so vivid that it obscures the present and governs our sensations, and drives our behavior and thinking.

Work with flashbacks requires the survivor to find a symbolic place of safety in their mind before the work begins, to feel safe in the room where you are working, and to feel secure in the therapeutic relationship. Begin by asking the survivor to visualize their safe place, and take them on a visualization journey from the room where you are working into that safe place. Get them to "feel" the textures, smells, and sensations of their safe place, to see themselves coming and going from their place of safety with ease.

Safety also demands that the survivor is in charge of the process, that they are empowered to say "no" if things feel too scary during the work. This is rooted in the very important insight that when trauma happens, the survivor will have lost control of their life in a deeply threatening and radical sort of way, and that the road to recovery involves achieving a flexible mastery again over oneself and the situations that life throws up.

The key to working with flashbacks is to have practiced a way of working with the survivor whereby they have learned to deeply relax when they are stimulated by scary thoughts and sensations. The relaxation work may need to go on for several sessions before tackling the flashbacks, and the survivor should practice relaxation and finding their place of safety at home.

Guidance

This work requires the survivor to find a symbolic place of safety in their mind before the work begins. To feel safe in the room where you are working. To feel secure in the therapeutic relationship. Ask the survivor to visualize their safe place, take them on a visualization journey from the room where you are working into that safe place. Get them to "feel" the textures, smells, and sensations of their safe place, to see themselves coming and going from their place of safety with ease.

> **Guidance**
>
> **Working with Flashbacks**
>
> 1. Establish a place of safety
> 2. Establish relaxation
> 3. "Play" with danger
> 4. Move from mild danger back to safety and relaxation
> 5. Bring flashback triggers into mind.
> 6. Breath into the sensations that flow from the trigger, locate those sensations in the body, slow them up
> 7. Move from flashback back to relaxation and safety
> 8. Move from the past (flashback) into the present
> 9. Be reminded "here is the present," "anchor yourself here," "come back to the present."
> 10. Using the present, yourself, the room, their place of safety as an anchor to the present

What then follows are sessions when the survivor is invited to bring milder aspects of the trauma to mind. The therapist follows intently what happens for the survivor physically and emotionally as this occurs, coaching them to breath into those physical and emotional responses. Through this the survivor is coached into noticing how the breath-work makes a subtle difference to how they experience the trauma, doing this until both therapist and survivor have a trusting grasp of the method. In this manner, the survivor is supported in breathing into what comes, what changes, and then reflecting. Next, the survivor is supported to use this breath-work, reflection, and relaxation to move to bringing into mind a more dangerous trigger, and then back through breath-work and reflection to relaxation and safety. Following this, they are invited to call to mind more of the scarier memories that trigger them and to work through them one by one.

If during the work with flashbacks, they begin to slip away into a dissociated place (a flashback is a form of dissociation) remind them to come back into the present. One has to walk an edge where the terrifying triggering memory can be invoked, and some degree of dissociation experienced, and uncomfortable sensations experienced, but the present remains intact. One has to work with a sense of progression staying relaxed and in control, moving away from overwhelming fear toward a place where the memory is intact and the trauma no longer has the power to overwhelm, to sting, or to harm. The ultimate goal is to move into a state of mind where he survivor can recall events with clarity in an emotionally balanced manner. This is almost a physiological process but accompanying it there often has to be examination and analysis of the emotions and thoughts thrown up by the process, "How did that feel then, how does it feel now?" and, "What thoughts did you have about yourself then, and what do you think now?".

Eye Movement Desensitization and Reprogramming (EMDR)

The final step in our work together work was EMDR (Eye Movement Desensitization and Reprogramming) EMDR is helpful if memories of the trauma are triggering, or avoidance of traumatic cues are interfering with life or emotional numbing is part of the everyday picture of life. EMDR will also resolve panic attacks and dissociation. EMDR was discovered almost by accident by the American psychologist Francine Shapiro. She noticed when she walked beside the park after a stressful morning with clients her negative emotions almost magically seemed to lift. When she paid attention to what was happening she realized it was the bars of light and shade playing into the eyes through the park railings that seemed to be making the difference. This embarked her on the discovery that became EMDR. What emerged is a treatment in which the therapist checks out the survivors' subjective feelings of distress felt in the body and mind in order to rate their intensity. A safe place is established in the survivor's mind, a place where they can go in their imagination if the procedure becomes too intense, and they are told they are in charge of the process and can bring it to a halt anytime they want if it feels too much. Once safety is established, the therapist invites the survivor to recall the central image of the trauma and then sweeps their hand across their field of vision. The survivor follows the hand movement with their eyes while allowing whatever arises in their mind simply to come, while watching the action at a distance, as if they were at a movie. The therapist pauses the eye movements periodically, checks in with the survivor and invites them to say whatever is coming into their mind and body. They then restart the procedure at that moment, return to the hand movements, and continue in this way until all the central features of the trauma and its associations have been run through. What happens is that the recall of the trauma combined with hand movements relieves the emotional and physiological charge of traumatic memories. This is a very simple explanation of a very detailed and carefully put together procedure that has dramatic results. Some therapists use EMDR as their primary way of treating trauma. My own preference is that it is used within an already established therapy relationship and as one of a range of different treatment approaches. Preparatory work with relaxation and breathing, and establishing real and symbolic safety needs to happen before EMDR can begin.

Learning Point

EMDR—Eye Movement Desensitization and Reprogramming

Uses a well-tested protocol to resolve the central aspects of the trauma that are most alarming and triggering to the survivor.

The treatment involves a treatment protocol used in conjunction with bilateral stimulation provided by eye movement (following the therapists hand moved from left to right across the field of vision) or an audio signal that sounds alternately in left and right ears or vibrating pulsars that pulse alternately in the left and right hand or tapping alternately left and right on the back of the hand or knees.

Various theories have been offered as to how EMDR does its magic. Fundamentally it is a form of bilateral (left and right) stimulation that can be provided by eye movement, sound, and tapping. What it seems to do is to free up the limbic brain to communicate with the higher cognitive brain, so the emotional response to trauma becomes more flexible, and traumatic memories are relieved and processed to the point where they take on the quality of ordinary recall, unpleasant but no longer capable of triggering a shocked physiological response.

Meeting the Need to Belong: Unravelling Inner and Outer Experience

Georgia already belonged but her preoccupation, moodiness, and irritation that were somewhat invisible to her in the middle of those moods kept people at bay. Trauma does this, it narrows our focus down to the imperatives of survival, so the things that enliven others seem paltry to us. Unravelling inner and outer experience is the ordinary work of psychotherapy but it is so important to make progress in recovery from trauma. We can see physiologically that cues such as loud noises, and sudden movements trigger startle responses and cause panic attacks and flashbacks in survivors, but almost surprisingly the link between these responses and the trauma may not be at all obvious to them. We see that making the link in a way that makes sense can ground the survivor and make them feel less panicked and mad. It can explain inner experience and offer ways of thinking how this plays out in circular ways in relationships that can create a more virtuous link between what is felt, how they react, and how this resonates for others. However, there are also some really subtle effects between inner and outer reality that can be utterly perplexing to a survivor and to their friends and families. For instance, an aid worker had an unusual and serious and physically unexplainable weakness in his ankle that we began to understand was a bodily memory of shame. He eventually recalled a repressed memory that he had trembled in utter terror at the bottom of the trench while a body guard had returned fire at some attackers while standing on his ankle to keep him pinned down and safe. Letting go of his shame undid his depression, allowed him to return to his work, undid the alienating effects of his unique experience, made him enjoy his friends again, and met his needs for belonging.

Needs for Esteem, and Self-Actualization

The need to hold a simultaneous inner and outer stance and help with linking is vital to the work. In Georgia's case, the trauma had heightened her sense of global responsibility, already well honed as a foreign correspondent, and images of the war in the news resonated with her sense of not having done enough to bring the war's atrocities to the eyes of the world. Once her basic safety needs had been met through psychological work, this troubling existential question needed to be explored and unravelled through weeks of therapy that linked her motivations to become a journalist with a proportionate grasp of what could be achieved, and a newly fashioned sense of a shared equity in human endeavor. Very often, as Dori Laub and Nanette Auerhahn (1993) have noticed powerful trauma linked life themes often drive survivors forward in the aftermath of extreme events, and one of the tasks of therapy and family and friendship surely is to open up and allow a space for that debate. It was in the corners of that discussion that Georgia recovered her sense of prestige and the life-affirming creativity of her career.

Transformation

Trauma undoes us, *and* it remakes us, this message flows through all accounts of trauma from Siegfried Sassoon *Memoirs of an Infantry Officer* (1930), through Victor Frankel *Man's Search for Meaning* (1946), Bruno Bettelheim *The Informed Heart* (1960), Primo Levi *The Drowned and the Saved* (1986), Brian Keenan *An Evil Cradling* (1991), Eric Lomax The Railway Man (1995) Murat Kurnaz *Five Years of My Life* (2008), Aziz BineBine *Tazamart* (2020), John Schlapobersky *When They Came for Me* (2021). Evil undoes us and we are remade in its wake, and what emerges is a subtle transformation in which our deeper connection with others in vulnerability comes to feel like an unshakeable conviction. The deeper meanings of life can spill into these spaces, almost numinous (filled with awe and wonder) in their intensity. Some people experience these in religious way, and prayer, contemplation, and meditation are deeply helpful practices for believers because they open up and nourish a reflective place within us (Woodcock 2001). On the other hand it can be that we are trapped in an identification with those who have been through the same or similar experience, even to the point of alienation from those whose lives seem untouched by trouble, although who are we to judge? But there are also processes that enable the singularity of experience to break through into a more general sense of deep and compassionate connection with others.

Groupwork and Transformation

Groupwork with survivors can create what John Schlapobersky (2016) describes as a relational matrix where our solitary experience is transformed. Psychotherapy with survivors has the same potential especially when the therapist has the capacity to move beyond the single therapist patient dynamic to invite the many symbolic witnesses on the sidelines to enter the therapeutic frame. Systemic Family Therapy is adept at this because throughout its work the wider family picture and our contexts of life are held in mind and threaded through therapeutic conversations, "What might so and so say, or think or feel or respond to what we're talking about or experiencing right now?" Families and friends can pick up these conversations too. A transformational conversation might wonder how each member of the family or friendship group would respond if they had been in the survivor's shoes, to how in turn they might respond to the thoughts, and feelings and conflicts in the survivor's mind. These aren't surefire ways of getting through because friends and family can be stubborn, rejecting and prefer not to see what we've experienced but more often than not there is more openness that might at first be imagined, particularly when the conversation is held in a safe and emotionally contained way.

Learning to Sit with Trauma and When to Respond

What emerges in all of this is learning when to sit with a loved one's trauma and when to respond. This can be agonizing when we want to help but the survivor isn't ready but is deeply troubled. Equally, we may not be ready, other family and friends may not want to participate. There can't be a blueprint here because we are all so different in temperament and life experience and trauma, however, the considerations that flow from Maslow's hierarchy of needs may help. Here are some principles.

1. There is no obligation at all for anyone to work through a trauma.
2. To work through trauma we need to feel safe enough to do the work. The paradox here is that trauma makes us feel dramatically unsafe but we need to be able to consider if our basic needs for safety have been met.
3. It probably isn't best to proceed with trauma work if the survivor's basic needs for safety are not in place.
4. Basic needs for safety have been met but the physiological and psychological aftermath of trauma are what is making the survivor feel unsafe, work may be considered—but the survivor must decide.
5. The survivor needs to decide to do the work, and to be in charge of its pace and direction.
6. Gentle work linking the trauma to feelings of panic and danger can help with realization of what drives the feelings of panic and other sensations of danger and can help ground the survivor.
7. At each stage consider how trauma is standing in the way of Maslow's needs being met.
8. Mostly each stage of Maslow's hierarchy of needs should be in place before moving onto the next.
9. Suggest links between trauma and physiological experience.
10. Suggest links between inner and outer experience

Mindfulness

In many ways mindfulness has been threaded through this chapter. Mindfulness is simply the practice of silently bringing awareness to our thoughts, feelings, and sensations in such a way that as soon as our mind starts to wander, or get fixated on a thought, feeling, or sensation we can bring it back to the present. This practice of mindful awareness is deeply encouraged by sitting in a relaxed manner and paying attention to or breathing in a very conscious way. It's very good to have a survivor practice mindfulness for some weeks before working with traumatic material. There is a danger here though that if we let our minds go free as mindfulness encourages, the thoughts and sensations that will jump into our consciousness are the worrying, anxious, and traumatic thoughts that we have struggled to keep at bay. So best to offer mindfulness with a health warning: its good for you, but if worrying thoughts come into your mind, go back to the breathing, count the breaths coming in, counting them going out up to ten, and begin again. If and when your thoughts drift, go back to the breath. It is a discipline that takes concentration but it reaps huge benefits. If the survivor finds it difficult to follow the discipline themselves there are some very good meditation apps that offer a guided course that gradually extends the meditation time from a few minutes up to as many as twenty-five. For a survivor sitting on their own prior to working through flashbacks five minutes a day is a good length of time to aim for.

Exercise

Mindfulness of Breathing Exercise

1. Sit in a quiet place in a chair with your feet on the floor, back upright and self-supported, head loosely balanced, chin slightly tucked in, shoulders low and relaxed, hands folded in the lap.
2. Breathe slowly into your abdomen, that place just below your belly button, place a hand there for a while to feel your tummy rise and fall.

---

3. Count the first breath in "One" and as you breath in slowly count one to seven.
4. Hold the breath for a second once its completely in and then let it go, counting one to ten.
5. Count the next breath in "Two" and so up to "Ten," following the method above, in for seven, out for ten.
6. When your thoughts wander, bring your attention back to your breath. If your thoughts have really wandered far so, your counting has been obliterated begin again at "One."
7. Be kind to yourself, your thoughts will wander.
8. Keep this up for five minutes.
9. Thank yourself and the practice as you finish your last breath, breathe out gratitude.

Summary

Each of the approaches outlined in this chapter is effective, they can be used together or alone and it depends on how the survivor responds and what choices they make that should guide what is done. For some, mindfulness opens the mind and body too abruptly. If that is so, use it carefully and cautiously, for instance, using a guided mindfulness script rather than leaving the survivor to use mindfulness on their own. For some working with flashbacks may be too triggering, in which case run through the method carefully and make sure that a place of safety is really well established. Indeed, work hard over several sessions just to establish a place of safety, there's no need to rush any of this work, work at the survivors pace always. EMDR may not work for some people, the recollected memories of the trauma can come back with vivid intensity and this requires a deep trust in the practitioner to hold a safe space. Indeed, EMDR is most effective when it is part of an ongoing therapeutic work where a good degree of therapeutic trust has been established. Work with linking as well as being deeply satisfying and explanatory can also be tricky if the links made rush ahead of what the survivor is ready to absorb, the key again is to follow the capacities of the survivor with sensitivity, and connection to their courage to survive. The above should not move us into work that is driven by technique, at best these are forms of awareness that one brings to work with trauma that become woven into our general approach as psychotherapists, part of the repertoire we draw on, which is set deeply into our relational approach, which knows that in the foreground, all this is about relationship making.

What We Can Do as Family and Friends

Consider all this together with the survivor and in your family/friendship circle, take turns to speak, listen, and reflect

Work out where we are on Maslow's hierarchy of needs. Where is the survivor, and what is blocking any progress up the hierarchy? How can we help?

Breathe into emotional and physical pain, watch how it changes; consider and reflect with a partner what is this hard path teaching us?

Create a place of safety together

Practice mindfulness of breathing and the body scan

Practice visualization and relaxation with each other

Just sit with things, no need to do a thing for a while

Use 7/11 breathing to calm panic attacks

Practice with the survivor and with each coming into the present when bad thoughts and sensations come

Take up exercise to burn off cortisol; invite someone to be your exercise guide and mentor, and you be theirs

References

Bettelheim, Bruno. 1960. *The Informed Heart*. New York: Free Press.

Binebine, Aziz. 2020. *Tazamart*. London: Haus Publishing.

Frankel, Victor. 1946. *Man's Search for Meaning*. London: Random House.

Kabatt-Zinn, Jon. 1990. *Full Catastrophe Living: How to Cope with Stress, Pain and Illness Using Mindfulness Meditation*. London: Piatkus.

Keenan, Brian. 1991. *An Evil Cradling*. London: Hutchinson.

Kurnaz, Murat. 2008. *Five Years of My Life*. London: Macmillan.

Laub, Dori, and Nanette Auerhahn. 1993. Knowing and Not Knowing Massive Psychic Trauma: Forms of Traumatic Memory. *International Journal of Psychoanalysis* 74: 287–302.

Levi, Primo. 1986. *The Drowned and the Saved*. London: Michael Joseph.

Lomax, Eric. 1995. *The Railway Man*. London: Vintage.

Rothschild, Babette. 2010. *8 Keys to Safe Trauma Recovery*. London: Norton.

Sassoon, Siegfried. 1930. *Memoirs of an Infantry Officer*. London: Faber & Faber.

Schlapobersky, John. 2016. *From the Couch to the Circle*. London: Routledge.

Schlapobersky, John. 2021. *When They Came for Me*. Oxford: Berghahn.

Woodcock, Jeremy. 2001. Trauma and Spirituality. In *Trauma: A Practitioners Guide to Counselling*, ed. Thom Spiers. London: Routledge.

8

Trauma and Death

When Michel was asked if he would help the overstretched emergency services recover bodies from the tsunami he was happy to help. However, happiness does not really encompass the farrago of emotions that compelled him to respond so readily. That morning he and his partner and their teenage son had been idly shopping in the stalls a few hundred meters from the beach when a powerful wash of water, uncanny for being so far inland, set up a panic in everyone around as it surged with unusual force. His partner was alarmed and Michel shouted to his son who was at another stall and who was light hearted and giddy in response to the event that was gathering momentum. He waded through the ankle-deep water, grabbed his son by the wrist, commanded his attention and they began to run just as a powerful rush of water began to tumble through the stalls pushing everything together like a concertina folding up. Behind them, a roar built with shocking intensity. Michel was terrified, and he ran like he had never run before across the main road that was filling with water with cars and tuk-tuks beginning to slew in

© The Author(s), under exclusive license to Springer Nature
Switzerland AG 2022
J. Woodcock, *Families and Individuals Living with Trauma*,
Palgrave Texts in Counselling and Psychotherapy,
https://doi.org/10.1007/978-3-030-79039-4_8

the powerful currents. Gasping for breath, they raced through the lobby of their hotel that was awash with water and up the stairs to the second floor where they watched in horror as water filled with debris surged past them, and everything between them and the beach was submerged under tumbling chaotic waves. They all survived although a number from the hotel who had been down on the beach died. Grateful for his own life and the life of his family, Michel bent to the task of collecting the dead. With two other volunteers, they lifted debris, hauled on limbs, and carried bodies of men and women and children in a blanket to a designated assembly point that by nightfall overflowed with the dead. That night he didn't sleep until the small hours. The following day, he was relieved that the volunteer recovery effort was stood down as trained rescuers and local government staff took over, and he and the family retreated to the capital to find a flight out just a few days later.

Nothing quite prepared Michel for the feelings that followed, the knowledge that he was utterly blessed to have survived, and the sense that he had come as close as a whisker to death. Whenever an image of the day passed through his mind, he shuddered inwardly. He was deeply imbued with a sense of social responsibility and this had compelled him to volunteer but his work that day had not discharged or diluted the panic he felt by his closeness to death. In the months that followed, although life back home in Europe was as usual as ever within him, he felt a deep sense of alienation. Colleagues at work were sweet and attentive to what he had experienced but to them, it was just a dramatic story, told a few times and then not quite forgotten but not revisited with the intensity that Michel experienced. And so Michel felt alienated, this brush with death had touched him viscerally, uncomfortably, and deeply.

The Singularity of Death

What Michel had experienced in vast measure was the absolute singularity of death. No death is ever the same, not even when like Michel, one encounters death many times in the same day. What came into Michel's mind constantly were the images of the dead people he had recovered, the shape of them curled into debris, half buried in mud and sand, pinned under beams, crushed and sliced open by the tumbled wreckage of buildings, the smell and the feel of them, and his empathy for men of his own age, children the same age as his son, toddlers, older men and women, each one a flashing image, and a feel in his hands and back and arms as he recalled the recovery. And the memories are not all fully intact, some distinct in every aspect, some blended but each one is also unique, and singular even when the images and sensations recalled blended together. It was the singularity of their deaths that struck him, although the overall situation that led to each of their deaths was the same, everyone was different, and it is this singular difference that has to be held in mind by anyone who lends support to someone who has experienced a traumatic death.

Every death is different whether traumatic or not and this is because each life is at the center of a web of connections and death severs those connections. It is as if each thread of that web amplifies the complexity and singularity of each death. No one person will have the same web that connects, and as Michel discovered in an almost uncanny way, this web of connections is written on people's faces and bodies, inscribed on their clothes, and on their possessions. Of course as he worked with each retrieval, he couldn't read each one accurately, even more so because he recovered people from so many different nationalities foreign to him. Nevertheless, he was acutely aware of the net of life that surrounded each person, even more so when he and his volunteer companions encountered groups of distressed relatives who gathered at the makeshift mortuaries that had been established.

Initially, the therapeutic work with Michel acknowledged the multiple nature of his trauma but it skimmed through his experience. The skimming was important, it didn't set out to minimize or overlook anything he had endured, it simply set out to capture an overview in the first session, to give him the experience of being heard, while keeping an ear out for details that required deeper enquiry. It also aimed at moving at his pace, holding the balance of what he wanted to open up, showing a fearless openness to whatever he brought, and the capacity to go into it with him when the moment was right. As ever, this required sensitivity to the cues he gave about what he could bear to bring and the capacity to lead the discussion into areas where he held back but that the therapist sensed it would be helpful to open up. What this led to was that Michel identified four deaths among the many he had witnessed that were outstandingly traumatic, these became the focus of the therapeutic work and the others, although no less important, became subsumed in that work as the traumatic charge of each of those was lessened. The work involved an exploration of the vivid sensations that formed Michel's memory of each of those deaths, each detail of their appearance, texture, smell, the physical sensations he experienced as he grappled with them; his thoughts and feelings, the detailed sensations he experienced in his body, and the emotions each one evoked in him, this included positive and negative memories, and the physical horror wrapped up in each encounter.

The Web of Life and Death

When this web of life and death is held in mind, it can help enormously to navigate conversations about traumatic death, whether these are conversations between a survivor and therapist or a survivor with their family, friends or other supportive companions. Naturally the direction of conversation and the topics covered are best negotiated in a self-consciously and mutually clear way between survivor and therapist or companion. Topics in the radial spokes of the web can be traced from the outside into the center to the depth and intensity that feels manageable. As the conversation progresses, one can also see how in the spiral of the web all the topics are interconnected, and as these connections unfold, the survivor can experience a profound sense of their traumatic experience being held in mind. It also means the conversation can be left in abeyance, and returned to when the opportunity is right, and more of the spiral can be navigated in a way that gives a sense of memory and continuity between sessions of discovery and healing (Fig. 8.1).

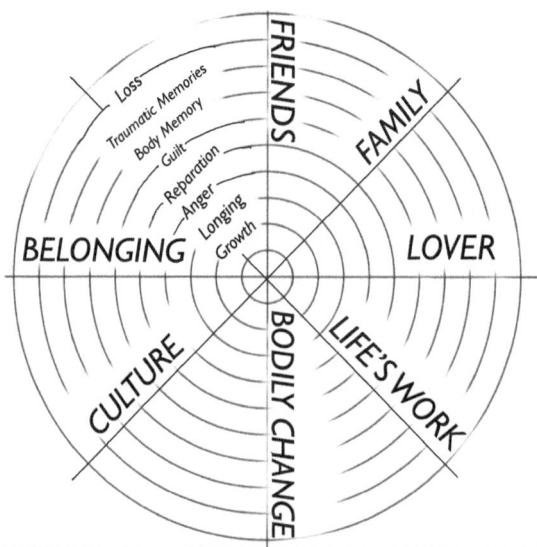

Fig. 8.1 The web of life and death

For instance, with Michel, starting in the innermost circle of the web, we tracked the losses he had experienced around that circle. Luckily objective losses were few in number but the symbolic losses were many for example his family were all equally affected as him, easy relations between them were lost, and their shared sense of belonging in a safe world was lost (family), friends who didn't appreciate quite how bad the experience was felt at a distance (friends). In the second inner-most circle, his traumatic memories flowed through thoughts about his family on the day (family), and he grieved that there was nothing in his immediate culture that anchored his experience of trauma, loss, and change (culture). His bodily memories ranged through the grip on his son's hand as they fled (family), the surging water around his legs, the massive shaking relief at finding his wife safe (lover), his deep sense of belonging to the small group of rescuers (belonging). His guilt and anger ranged at friends who were now distant because they didn't seem to fully understand (friends; belonging), his life work that now seemed trivial in comparison to the multitude of death he had witnessed (life's work), the sense that life back in Europe seemed materialistic and shallow (culture; belonging). Reparation and growth emerged as he allowed his cultural landmarks to expand to encompass his experience, and he began to feel a deeper citizen of the world (culture), this gave him a deeper sense of belonging (belonging), which he shared with family and invited friends (family; friends) into through fundraising activities he entered into to raise money for devastated communities in Sri Lanka.

The Need to Remember and the Wish to Forget

Something that will accompany many conversations about traumatic death is the tension between what has been described as the need to remember and the wish to forget. For instance, when Emina escaped the terrible war in Bosnia in the 1990's that had seemingly confounded every western power, she felt ruined by grief for her father, a teacher and intellectual, who had been executed by the other warring parties. Her last memories of him were agonizing, as he was dragged away from their home, and then another after frantic days when she had discovered him imprisoned behind the mesh of camp, freezing cold, inadequately clothed, bleeding and bruised, and hungry, and she was hustled and bullied and dragged away from the fence and then news of his death, inexplicable that a man as gentle as he should have been executed. On one occasion seeking a glimmer of hope into her future I asked her if she possessed anything that represented her lost homeland and she said, "Yes, a handful of soil from my father's grave." In some ways that encounter summarizes the need to remember and the wish to forget. What stands out is her need to remember her father but the enormous pain she felt when she called him to mind. She really did want to remember him but the pain that was evoked by her recollections of him during his arrest and the prison camp was so intense that she just could not grieve him properly.

Learning Point

Traumatic Grief

Shock and Numbness: this response very often follows loss, as if to survive the initial shock of the loss, the grieving person becomes numb and shut down

Disorganization and Despair: apathy, anger, despair, and hopelessness come and go with degrees of acceptance but deeper acceptance of loss is constantly interrupted by feelings of shocking memories of the death, by feelings of remorse and guilt that they couldn't protect the dead person or part from them in a loving way

Yearning and Searching: this response calls up many feelings, including sadness, anger, and anxiety. There is longing for the lost person and a wish for them to return to fill the empty spaces created by their death. In traumatic grief, as thoughts and memories of the dead person come, they are punctuated by intense recollections of horror that drive them back into shock and numbness alternated with anger, anxiety, and intense sadness

Reorganization and Recovery: there is no new normal, until the traumatic memories that form an impenetrable barrier to sustained positive memories of the lost person can be laid to rest. Once this is achieved the intense feelings of sadness, anger, and despair diminish. Positive memories of the lost person increase. Physical energy and vitality begin to return

In order to grieve, we feel the shock of death so deeply that it is difficult to believe that they are gone, we think almost irrationally how could they subject us to such pain by leaving us? But in order to grieve, we need to bring the lost person into mind, and of course, this is ordinarily painful, often deeply, sharply, and terribly hard to bear and yet this is the work of grief, to recall and to savor memories however painful, to pine for the person lost, to feel the sting of regret, to wish we could have done things better. In these ways, we experience the loss deeply and fully. Sometimes we find ourselves completely disorganized and muddled forgetting the most obvious things. Life feels as if we are on a tilting ship far out at sea, nothing is in its place, our hands can't find the things they need. Important aspects of the relationship come back into our mind, some most difficult to recollect because of the acutely felt failures in the relationship, some magically restorative when for moments the person who has died resides in our mind as if they are still alive, remembered, and imagined conversations take place, and we circulate through these spaces in our mind and in the actual spaces of our life the lost person physically occupied. And gradually, in normal grief, although there is no real normal, every grief is different, we arrive at a place of acceptance.

For Emina, there could be no place of acceptance, seemingly every time an ordinary memory came into her thoughts, her mind recoiled back to their traumatic parting. Here a distinction is made between thought and mind, and this distinction is important because there are times during traumatic re-experiencing when our thoughts are seemingly out of control and our mind has a life of its own. The truth is that when we pay our mind attention, we discover it does very often do its own thing. When life is good we are content for our mind to do its thing and we bring concentration to our fluctuating awareness and navigate our thoughts and emotions, but when we are in tumult, our mind may seem completely out of control with such a life of its own that drives our thoughts and emotions in ways that feel crazy, so that even the greatest efforts of concentration are overwhelmed. The question here was how to help Emina escape from the narrow hell where she found herself, could she fully grieve, and open up into the wide fields of happy memories she had of her father?

How to Help with Deeply Traumatic Grief

The first thing to acknowledge with a grief as powerful as Emina's is how the traumatic memories form an almost impenetrable roadblock which mean that sustained positive memories of the lost person cannot be reached. When working with the web of life and death, no sooner does a thought or memory come to mind than this triggers terrible memories that crowd out happy recollections. Body work is the place to start, calming the body's limbic responses, breath-work to calm, accompanied with sustained attention to how the body responds when a memory or fragment comes into mind, calling back into the present moment if a fugue state threatens to sweep them away and alongside this being carefully, and accurately attentive and emotionally available and led by them as to what they can tolerate. Through this careful work slowly enabling their window of tolerance to open until they reach the point where the whole traumatic narrative can be recalled without triggering a flight into a shocked fugue-like limbic response.

Guidance

Fugue States

A fugue state is best described as a state of mind when traumatic recollections are so strong that they block out our sense of being in the present. It is a powerful dissociated state of mind. Sometimes during a fugue state, the trauma seems so real that aspects of it are re-enacted. Responses can be powerful with shocked, or fearful, or spaced out facial expressions, physical gestures, and irregular panicked breathing.

Knowing that a fugue state might happen plan with the survivor, how you will respond as a helper. For instance, as it begins to occur, call the survivor back into the present, remind them you are here with them, coach them back into good breathing, invite them to focus on things in the room, encourage them back.

Whether to Seal off Memories or Work with Them

In work with trauma, there is a valuable debate about whether one works with traumatic memory or helps the survivor to sustain calm by sealing off memories of the traumatic event. However, with a survivor of a traumatic death, that debate leans heavily in the direction of work with the traumatic memory, because to seal off trauma is to cut off memory of their loved one, and the road back to positive memories has to pass through the fire of traumatic loss.

Guidance

Creating a Healthy Pattern of Sleep

Stay away from caffeine based drinks such as tea, and coffee and cheese or sugary foods from the afternoon until bedtime

Bed only for sleeping or cuddles or sex, get up to do anything else

Stay away from TV, computers, tablets, smartphones in at least the last two hours before bedtime, if possible for longer

A little light reading if that makes you sleepy, but not on a device

Follow this with breath work, stretching and relaxation, a warm bath or a shower

Set the alarm for the same time everyday and get up no matter how bad your sleep has been

Go to bed at the same time every day

No sleeping or naps during the day

Learning Point

The Reality Principle

Reality can be hard to bear but reality is best as long as it can tolerated	When traumatized we may need to give up the defenses we put in place to protect us from traumatic memory carefully and gradually and only when our limbic system can tolerate reality
	Working with the *window of tolerance* is a fine way of gradually allowing reality in

---

Sleep

As Emina began to gain control of her bodily responses through careful body work in twice weekly sessions, she reported how she was beginning to sleep better. We worked on her dreams that often involved terrible scenes that woke her in a panic. She did bodywork before bedtime, breathing and stretching, staying away from stimulants that included drinks with caffeine, sugary food, and cheese, and late evening television and tablets and phone. For several months, she laughed that she was living like a nun, but this work took hold, and she began to calm. The work on her dreams involved her bringing the dreams that troubled her allowing her to "breathe into them so she calmed, while we untangled their meaning, and she created alternative endings, where she wasn't horribly out of control but was able to keep a reflexive working eye on herself, offering thoughts and insights, accompanying herself through the dream landscape as a reflexive presence sometimes changing the ending of a dream when it was intolerable but mostly working with the reality principle, this principle being that it is most favorable to arrive at a point where one can tolerate reality rather than changing or denying it, but knowing one gets to such a reckoning by degrees and that our defenses against reality have to be respected, and this fits with the idea of a window of tolerance. Sometimes reality is too much to tolerate, but gradually with help, and warmth, and support it can gradually be let in. And there's no need to rush. And so it was with Emina. In the early days she woke very often in a panic and it was suggested she have a talisman she could keep under her pillow to reach for in the night. For her talisman, she chose a piece of wood she had found on a wood-land walk, whittled and smoothed by a friend, we invested it with safe thoughts, she breathed into it, counted her breath until she calmed. It was an object that brought her into the now, allowed her to practice calm and that she could hold as she slipped back into sleep. There were nights when she hardly slept at all but eventually, it did get better, and she followed the advice to wake at the same time every day, even at its worst, because that was the best way to establish and hold a good pattern of sleep.

Guidance

Working with dreams

Invest in a talisman imbued with safe and positive thoughts and feelings to reach for and hold during nightmares	Unpack the symbolic meanings of dreams
Use breath work to calm	Work on alternative endings to horrible dreams not ultimately as an end in itself (see reality principle) but as a way of creating a calm, reflexive observing self, that can accompany oneself through dreams and in the dead of night

Alienation

One of the hardest and almost invisible things to bear when death has been traumatic is the sense of alienation that engulfs survivors. Alienation is the powerful sense that we are cut off from ordinary life, a sense that life goes on outside of us as if through a plate glass window, the apprehension that we have experiences, feelings, and weird physical sensations that other people could never understand. For survivors with traumatic grief, this can show itself as the belief that our traumatic memories are too intense, unusual, bizarre, shocking, and toxic to be revealed and shared. The best antidote to alienation is to be invited back into life by people who can really hear the story with all its edges, emotional resonances, bizarre cul-de-sacs, toxic thoughts and feelings, and there is no doubt this is hard work to do, it needs a strong and loving heart and mind, and support for those who listen. Equally, alienation can be amazingly lessened when the survivors are enabled to share their experience with other survivors. Survivors have said things in groups like, "I never thought I would find or feel understood by another person who had been through the things that I experienced."

The Pathway Toward Recovery

The pathway toward recovery from experiences as shocking as the ones described in this chapter does not come easily. No death is easy to mourn, the sense of a gap torn into the fabric of one's life, and threads cut off will be harder when death has been unexpected, even more so when it happens before time through accident, disaster, warfare, or atrocities. There are paths toward recovery though, this chapter has described a few ways in detail that allow a therapist or the survivor's companions to lend their help. Yet we have to recognize that although grief lessens, mourning never truly ends, nor can it when we survive with our memories, loss will be felt years and years later. The hope here is that the alienation of traumatic death can be overcome with therapeutic attention, with the company of people who can listen and empathically enter the space of suffering, who have the skill to relax, restore sleep, navigate nightmares, tackle fugue states. Other chapters describe other ways that are part of this recovery, every path will be different. And Emina did come through, a simple but powerful ritual helped. One day, she took the bag of earth she had scraped from her father's grave back in her homeland and she mixed it with the earth in a garden in the new city where she lived, and she planted a climbing plant. Both survive.

What We Can Do as Family and Friends

Consider all this together with the survivor and in your family/friendship circle, take turns to speak, listen, and reflect

What are our beliefs, myths, assumptions, and hopes about grief and mourning and loss and change and death?

How do we allow grief to take its course, support the survivor's grief, and support each other's grief, when we all grieve differently?

Invite absent friends and family members to join us in our minds today. What would they say about all these questions (above and below) if they were here? Each of us will hold a different version of their voice. Can we be curious about what comes forth as we bring all those rich and varied voices together?

Talk about losses, allow space for them daily.

Find or create a daily ritual to represent loss.

Consider how to hold in mind the wish to remember and the need to forget.

Map out loss and change on the wheel of life and death

Talk about dreams; invite someone to be your dream guide and mentor, and you be theirs.

Find a safe object or talisman for nightmares.

Work on good endings for scary dreams.

Support a healthy pattern of sleep, the key is to get up at the same time every day.

9

Social Systems That Promote Attachment Versus Systems That Create Trauma

This chapter may seem of more concern for the professional reader, but it contains a lot for survivors and for family and friends because this is a chapter about searching for and establishing resilience in the very framework of our lives, and challenging situations that undermine us and can create the preconditions for trauma.

Poverty and Trauma

When a reckoning is made of the incidence of trauma across the globe the links between poverty and economic disadvantage are all too apparent. Consider for example the impact of Corona Virus. Although we may be all too familiar with its deadly toll in Europe and the United States, the effects in relatively poorer countries have been vivid and deadly. A powerful example of this is provided by the novelist Arundhati Roy writing in the Financial Times (2020) about the situation in India:

© The Author(s), under exclusive license to Springer Nature
Switzerland AG 2022
J. Woodcock, *Families and Individuals Living with Trauma*,
Palgrave Texts in Counselling and Psychotherapy,
https://doi.org/10.1007/978-3-030-79039-4_9

As an appalled world watched, India revealed herself in all her shame
— her brutal, structural, social and economic inequality, her callous indifference to suffering. The lockdown worked like a chemical experiment
that suddenly illuminated hidden things. As shops, restaurants, factories
and the construction industry shut down, as the wealthy and the middle
classes enclosed themselves in gated colonies, our towns and megacities
began to extrude their working-class citizens — their migrant workers —
like so much unwanted accrual. Many driven out by their employers and
landlords, millions of impoverished, hungry, thirsty people, young and
old, men, women, children, sick people, blind people, disabled people,
with nowhere else to go, with no public transport in sight, began a long
march home to their villages. They walked for days, towards Badaun,
Agra, Azamgarh, Aligarh, Lucknow, Gorakhpur — hundreds of kilome-
tres away. Some died on the way. Our towns and megacities began to
extrude their working-class citizens like so much unwanted accrual. They
knew they were going home potentially to slow starvation. Perhaps they
even knew they could be carrying the virus with them, and would infect
their families, their parents and grandparents back home, but they desper-
ately needed a shred of familiarity, shelter and dignity, as well as food, if
not love. As they walked, some were beaten brutally and humiliated by
the police, who were charged with strictly enforcing the curfew. Young
men were made to crouch and frog jump down the highway. Outside
the town of Bareilly, one group was herded together and hosed down
with chemical spray. A few days later, worried that the fleeing population
would spread the virus to villages, the government sealed state borders
even for walkers. People who had been walking for days were stopped
and forced to return to camps in the cities they had just been forced to
leave. Among older people it evoked memories of the population transfer
of 1947, when India was divided and Pakistan was born. Except that this
current exodus was driven by class divisions, not religion. Even still, these
were not India's poorest people. These were people who had (at least until
now) work in the city and homes to return to. The jobless, the homeless and the despairing remained where they were, in the cities as well as
the countryside, where deep distress was growing long before this tragedy
occurred.

These are prophetic words, an unwavering eye that gazes at the seeming
caprice of inequality. What is shocking about this description is a

consciousness of the fact that India has many resources and yet those are dramatically tilted away from the poor. The poor and dispossessed across the globe have suffered similar fates in the face of the global pandemic. The uncomfortable truth is that the same is true in wealthy countries like our own. In the United Kingdom, although it was clear that age was the clearest determinant of vulnerability, the burden of death fell on those with least resources. For instance, the Health Foundation (2020) reported that, "Of the 10 local areas in Great Britain with the highest death rates from COVID-19, half of them are from the poorest 30% of local authorities and Britain's poorest communities are facing a double whammy of health and financial hardship as a result of the COVID-19 pandemic and the responses to it." This was echoed by researchers writing in the Journal of Epidemiology and Community Health "Historically, pandemics have been experienced unequally with higher rates of infection and mortality among the most disadvantaged communities— particularly in more socially unequal countries. Emerging evidence from a variety of countries suggests that these inequalities are being mirrored today in the COVID-19 pandemic." Similar scenes have been described by researchers in the United States, for example, the Brookings Institute wrote: "COVID-19 has been described as a heat seeking missile speeding toward the most vulnerable in society. The Lancet reported (2020), "Confirming existing disparities, within New York City and other urban centres, African American and other communities of colour have been especially affected by the COVID-10 pandemic." That metaphor applies not just to the vulnerable in the rich world; the vulnerable in the rest of the world are not more immune. They may actually be easier targets."

What Could Be More Natural Than a Natural Disaster

What the pandemic illustrated rather horribly is that when disaster strikes those most vulnerable are already weakened by poor housing, education, healthcare, employment, access to services, work environment, and food. These facts pertain not only in pandemics but in natural disasters. This is striking because what could be more natural than a natural disaster? And yet when the Brookings Institute in 2017 surveyed the effects of hurricanes on the United States, it showed that the result of severe hurricanes result is that the more affluent migrate out of disaster hit zones leaving the poor behind (Brookings Institute 2017). These facts are compounded across the globe, for instance, when Stephanie Hallegatte (2020) surveyed the situation with her colleagues they discovered that it is the poor who settle into areas prone to flooding because these are vacated by those who are more wealthy and house and land prices fall making them attractive to people who are impoverished. Furthermore, often these places are close to industrial areas or tracts of farmland where there are jobs, as well as to schools and healthcare, and so poorer people take the risk of settling these places to gain access to social benefits.

Even when war impacts a whole population it is the poor who suffer disproportionately. Those with the means escape arrive by air into countries of refuge, while those without means are displaced across international boundaries into refugee camps and areas of temporary settlement or are forced to make perilous journeys. In addition, as described by Joanna Macrae and Anthony Zwi (1992) war and natural disaster lead to radical impoverishment, it is striking that in a world where there are the resources to adequately nourish everyone desperate famine situations occur in countries where there is warfare, sometimes occurring because farming and infrastructure are so destroyed that food cannot be grown and distributed, and often because famine is used as a means of war, to deplete an undermine enemy populations.

These are brutally stark examples of the potent mix of poverty and trauma and the need for policy approaches that embody social justice to be embodied in any approach to trauma. Furthermore, historical examples abound of how trauma resonates down through the generations. The call for social justice at the heart of the Black Lives Matter is a vivid example of this. The trauma of slavery is hard to imagine, of lives radically disrupted, the fact that the brutal plunder of people from West and their transportation into slavery was so widespread in Europe and the United States, that slave labor was a massive engine of economic power demonstrate how radical inequality flourishes when people are dehumanized, and the consequences of this resonate down the generations into the present day in the way that racism has been structured into the landscape of inequality in the United States and Europe. It is not an accident that in Britain and the United States, the pandemic has impacted most brutally on people of color. Policy debates have puzzled at the reasons why this should be so and yet what is most stark is that racism and inequality are the culprits yet again because if you are a person of color generations of discrimination mean that you are more likely to be poorer, to live in more crowded accommodation where transmission of the virus is more likely, to have work in areas that expose you to greater risk, such as less protected ancillary roles in the health service, or to be on the frontline in public transport and other service industries.

Gender and Trauma

Yet another determinant of trauma is gender. Just in summarizing the statistics of the effect of natural disaster and warfare Caroline Criado Perez writes (2019), "It's not the disaster that kills you" it is actually the gendered consequences of disaster. For instance, in a pandemic being the one who has the greater caretaking role and therefore exposure to infection. The fact that domestic violence breaks out when conflict breaks out and this was borne out in the conflict in Bosnia, in the Rwandan genocide and the civil war in Sierra Leone. In her compelling book that disaggregates the occurrence of effects on women from the general statistics of the effects of life on us all, she points out, when women are no longer overlooked in the analysis, the effects on women of war and disaster are massively skewed against them. The chilling point here is that in the wars that have swept the globe since the signing of the UN Declaration on Human Rights in 1948, the majority of deaths have been civilian, and among those, a massive proportion have been women. What Perez points out is that caretaking, fetching water, and husbandry that are typically women's responsibilities both place them at huge risk, and these are routinely overlooked when health and disaster management strategies are put in place, and because they have not seen the bad effects on women are further amplified.

Social Systems That Promote Attachment vs. Systems That Create Trauma

What each of these examples starkly illustrates is that there are social systems that promote trauma and there are social systems that ameliorate or lessen it. Furthermore, what is proposed here is that when social systems promote attachment, they create resilience to trauma, and when social systems do not value attachment and undermine opportunities to promote and sustain it, they promote the conditions where trauma flourishes.

Learning Point

Social systems that promote attachment look like this:

- There is good healthcare, and good access to healthcare

- There is good parental leave when children are born

- Housing has proportions that are generous enough to enable people space for privacy and mixing

---

- There is generous sickness entitlement

- Housing design is sympathetic to people's need to mix and have recreational opportunities within walking distance of home

- There is generous holiday entitlement

- Education promotes relational learning from early years on

- Part-time and flexible working arrangements are available and pay and career development are sufficient to allow this to happen without penalizing people making these choices

- Care of the sick, infirm and elderly is imbued with relational values

Social systems that promote attachment first and foremost value attachment. This was true even before attachment was formalized into theory by John Bowlby and others in the 1960s (Bowlby 1969, 1973). Instances of this are the work that Anna Freud (1966) did with child survivors of the holocaust; she understood that what had made them resilient was being in a gang, being attached to each other, and she allowed these gangs to survive when the children were later cared for in children's homes (Freud 1966). This was also true of the International Children's Villages set up to care for displaced children after the war, children who had been displaced and travelled together were allowed to live together, as is beautifully illustrated in Ian Serrallier's wonderful story, *The Silver Sword (1956)*. These of course are small social systems where benign adults tolerated the oddities of children's behavior that had developed as strategies for survival such as mistrust of authority, thieving, ganging up against outsiders, including the carers themselves, while at the same time they offered empathic and attuned attention. What is true in each of these situations and true also of children who escape situations of abuse and oppression is that they adapt their attachment strategies in order to survive, and the younger that children are when these survival strategies start the more entrenched into their personality they become (Crittenden 2008). This final point bears out a truth, which is that attachment patterns are not something separate to a person that can be tinkered with, attachment is intrinsic to our personalities, and this is why social systems that promote attachment are so valuable to the overall well-being of individuals *and* society at large.

Relational Learning

Relational learning simply means all forms of learning that place the relationship at the heart of their endeavors. This may be overt such as a school having lessons about anti-bullying and adolescent relationships, and for instance, placing relationship at the center of teaching about sex, so less on biology, which is important, but more on tenderness, protection, excitement, fun, and playfulness, which are all aspects of good relationships. Relational learning is also learned through seeing relationships at work, where education is geared in ways that promote collaboration rather than competition, where group learning is seen as the way forward rather than undue emphasis on individual success, where teachers interact with students in ways that are empathic and attentive and where authority is invested in relationship.

Social systems That Work Against Attachment Cause Trauma

It is possible even now that we are just emerging from the depredations of early capitalism, which sucked vast populations of people displaced off the land because of the enclosures act into the cities and imposed on them work practices that worked against family life, health and well-being. Social systems that work against attachment are characterized by the manner in which people are divided, and objectified and ultimately dehumanized. Simply put, in very stratified societies where there is a vast gulf between what the top earners receive and what those who earn least, there is an impulse for this to be justified through dehuman-ization—the sense being that one is better and deserving when others are lesser and undeserving. Such a sensibility only works because one is cut-off in some way from an open, connected and relational emotional response to the lived situation of people who as a consequence suffer lives of deprivation. This dynamic is revealed in microcosm in boarding school life as described by Nick Duffell and Thurstine Bassett (2016), in which children as young as eight are left at preparatory school and left to manage their feelings of abandonment by walling off painful sensations and covering them up with a mixture of group loyalty and vicious competitive spirit in which one cannot afford to show weak-ness, and where outsiders of the narrow economically privileged and yet emotionally pinched life of the school and its wider class are berated and scapegoated as a hedge against one's own desperate feelings. These experiences create what George Orwell (1969) described as a subaltern class, equipped to dominate and rule because they have imbued into them a belief in their innate superiority and by default the inferiority of people subject to their authority. In effect this was a traumatized class that exported trauma to the far corners of the world through the colonial endeavors of the British Empire.

Learning Point

Social systems that work against attachment look like this:

- There is poor healthcare, and access to healthcare is rationed and discriminatory

- There is little or no entitlement to parental leave

- People have to work full-time and beyond to make ends meet

- Cramped housing has too little room for privacy and open space for relaxed living

---

- There is little entitlement to sickness benefits so people have to make hard choices about their economic well-being versus their health

- Education promotes individual values and competitive learning

- There is little holiday entitlement so family and friends have fewer opportunities for prolonged periods of relationship ease and relaxation

- Care of the sick, infirm and elderly are deprived of resources and continuity of care is fragmented

Family Violence and Trauma

By definition, to be attached means to be accurately attentive to the emotional needs of others. Family violence emerges in social systems that do not value attachment, where men, most often believe they have a right to behave in ways that are violent, coercive, and controlling. For reasons to do with patriarchal histories lost in the mists of time men have almost habitually internalized a sense of their superiority over women. These are not abstract facts but the lived reality of centuries and played out in often gross but also the most subtle interactions in society today, for instance, where boys receive much greater attention in mixed science and mathematics classes. What is being conveyed is not something equal and relational but a subtle set of values that deform our ability to relate as equals and that is what is at the base of degraded relationships. These same patterns get played out in family violence that move from subtle to overt and violent control as Pat Craven describes in *Living with the Dominator* (2008), and where sometimes, to their cost women find that they have internalized a set of values that are inimical to their own well-being, in which they too uphold the superiority of men and their own objectification as stupid, or provocative and deserving of rejection or violence. One can also conjecture that a social system that is depriving and discriminatory and conveys powerful messages that people are not to be valued sets up the conditions whereby emotional attachments within families and between people are strained to the utmost. Good attachment offers intimacy, and if intimacy is defined as the capacity to meet another with reciprocal vulnerability and tenderness, with an open heart and mind, family violence is the opposite of that.

It seems then that social systems that make emotional attachment difficult to achieve are social systems that cause trauma. The causal link works in two directions: we saw optimal attachment described in Chapter 5, and this was contrasted with attachments that are strained in the direction of watchfulness when there is fear of the parental figure, and the child's survival strategy is to depress their own attachment demands and keep a look out, and we saw an almost opposite strategy when the parent is neglectful and emotionally absent, when the child's survival strategy is to demand to be noticed. What becomes habitually present in both of these forms of attachment is a form of splitting, whereby vulnerable emotions are repressed and denied in favor either of some degree of coercive control, where one puts oneself in charge of getting one's needs met, rather than it being truly open and reciprocal relationship or where one represses one's conscious need for connection and affection and puts the other in charge of stepping forward to meet those needs, again a strategy that is not truly open or reciprocal. These are stark examples of course, and the subtlety of attachment theory is that it understands these ways of behaving as existing on a continuum, and also that these habitual ways of behaving in intimate relationships are deeply interwoven with our personalities, so none is ever exactly the same. The thing is that societies also behave in these ways, social systems split off emotions from situations or people are seen or imagined as denuded of emotion, or when emotion is revealed, it is conceptualized as irrational and off the point, or even more worryingly the emotions of others are not equated with our own, in other words, there is deemed to be no commensurability between what *we* feel and what *they* feel. This sort of splitting justifies why others in society, often poorer, less well educated, or people of color, or foreign in some way may be treated differently to ourselves. We have also seen that in traumatic situations, we behave in these ways, we split off our feelings because they are so terrifying and overwhelming, and possibly likely to overwhelm our capacity to do whatever it is, we need to do to survive. In at least one form of post-traumatic stress disorder this splitting occurs habitually because trauma has become a bodily memory that continually revisits, and we split away from those memories because they threaten to overwhelm us again and again, this is part of the underlying structure of dissociation.

Learning Point

Splitting Explained

Basically—when emotions or situations are so unbearably powerful we push them out of mind

Psychological—when an emotional vulnerability is so overwhelming it is denied and pushed out of mind

Attachment—when a need is so raw we cannot dare to show it or we even fear to show it

Trauma—when terror is so powerful we cannot hold it in our mind

---

Society also splits itself off from emotions that threaten to overwhelm. For instance, it can be conjectured that immigration policy keeps refugees out because they are so infected with the overwhelmingly horrible experiences that we would rather not have anything to do with them. Or even more locally, when poor families cannot afford to feed their children, it can be unbearable to think about their needs and to offer remedies in a rational, joined up, and compassionate way.

Attachment as Tenderness

Another word for attachment might be tenderness. Tenderness implies actions that are modulated kindness and with fellow feeling, where there is a focus that is attentive, attuned and in step with the needs of the other person, balanced about how it is offered, so not intrusive nor ineffective because too tentative, and yet reciprocal because the human dimension is present where there is a consciousness that nothing separates oneself from the other person, that one very easily could be in that place of need. The question that flows from this is how can social systems promote attachment and tenderness? It almost seems an almost absurd proposal and yet the argument here is that when attachment is placed at the heart of social systems, this provides protection against trauma and the intergenerational transmission of trauma.

Social Systems Geared Toward Attachment

Social systems that are geared toward attachment set out to create the optimal conditions where attachment and tenderness can thrive, where home and work and leisure and housing and neighborhood are set up on a human scale, that values our connection to each other, where measures constantly evolve to strengthen communities, where there is a deep recognition that everyone has to thrive, there is no splitting, no them and us and where each child's attachment to its parents or caregivers and work is geared toward to that value that and no one has to struggle on wages that are so low that they have to compromise caring in order to work, and where social dis-eases like gender violence are confronted through education that values the chances of both genders.

Attachment, Violence, and Trauma

Violence is the shadow that lurks under here. It would seem that we have to give way to its primal qualities, that to deny that is an intrinsic quality of humanness is to be hopelessly idealistic, and to imagine we can live in societies where attachment and tenderness are the guiding principles is utterly foolish. However, at the heart of an understanding of trauma is the realization that the urge to violence emerges out of a limbic system that is set up to protract us from harm, and that one of the greatest social harms is severe and enduring economic deprivation, and this creates and perpetuates violence: structural violence that leads me to accumulate as protection and therefore deprives you because resources are limited. Prisons across the world are filled with men who have limbic systems that are primed toward violent accumulation and violent self-protection, and yet there is clear evidence emerging as Nina Papali (2019) describes that multi-modal therapeutic interventions that are geared toward promoting staying in relationship and de-tuning violent, limbic-driven responses can be highly effective. Often the philosophical idea that underpins our hopelessness about violence is the Augustinian-Christian notion that we are "born bad" (Boyce 2016), and yet although this idea has deeply infiltrated law and public policy in Europe and the United States, there is equal evidence that we aren't born bad at all, we're just born and that cultural and social determinates are the prime drivers that shape us. Of course in Europe and the United States, one of those determinates will be the notion that we are born bad, and some of us are born so particularly bad that there's nothing that can be done to help or change us for the better, and this underpins a laissez-faire attitude to public policy, that pushes toward the notion that we are all individuals who are entirely responsible for our own fate, a particularly nice view from the standpoint of privilege, but less inviting but nevertheless equally likely to be believed by those who have very little. By contrast, attachment thinking suggests the opposite, the way forward is through connection not individualism, and furthermore, there's good evidence, as revealed in Chapter 3 that's the way our brain, and nervous system and physiology are set up, if we would listen.

Resilience to Trauma

When we stay in relationship with others we are most resilient to trauma. It is intrinsic to trauma that it strains and attacks our capacity to relate because the limbic system set up to protect us fires up in ways that sacrifice the higher functions of attachment in order to look after ourselves as a basic physiological entity and that after trauma, and repeated re-traumatization caused by the limbic system by staying on self-protective high alert, our capacity to relate is compromised. However, if we can simultaneously calm the limbic system and stay in relationship (and a calm limbic system really helps us stay in relationship), our chances of a good ongoing life are greatly enhanced. What this points toward is that the key to resilience at its most simple is triangular: a calm limbic system, leading to a capacity for relationship, underpinned by social systems that promote relationship. And this is circular because when social systems support relationship, they understand intrinsically and promote the conditions where calm connection can thrive.

Frameworks for Social Protection Are Frameworks for Self Protection

The final point to be made is that frameworks for self-protection are frameworks for social protection. For instance, in disaster situations when women can bathe and go to the toilet without being predated on this enhances their capacity to be reciprocally caring. When my neighbor's child is being properly fed, it means we and our children can meet as equals and look after each other when disaster strikes. When there is a pandemic neighbor networks of care and support are enormously important.

What We Can Do as Family and Friends

Consider all this together with the survivor and in your family/friendship circle, take turns to speak, listen, and reflect
Practice tenderness
Consider, what is the practice of equality?
Stand up for yourself, and your community.
Consider, what are the limits of my tolerance, and what then?
Practice staying in relationship even when it's hard; use attunement and listening skills.
Support friends, neighbors, community; invite someone to be your neighbors and community mentor, and you be theirs.
Practice relational learning, where relationships are at the heart of how we learn.

Get hold of a little book on non-violent communication, practice as a group; understand non-violence is really strong.

Find out how things join up, be a connected person, family, friendship circle.

When someone expresses pain, don't leap into action, tune in, empathize, hear how it feels (from Wayland Myers [1998] *Non-Violent Communication: The Basics as I Know and Use Them*. Encinitas, CA: Wayland Myers Books).

References

Bowlby, John. 1969. *Attachment: Attachment and Loss* (vol. 1) (2nd ed.). New York: Basic Books.

Bowlby, John. 1973. *Separation: Anxiety & Anger*. Attachment and Loss (vol. 2) (International psycho-analytical library no. 95). London: Hogarth Press.

Boyce, James. 2016. *Born Bad: Original Sin and the Making of the Western Mind*. London: SPCK.

Brookings Institute. 2017. https://www.brookings.edu/blog/social-mobility-memos/2017/09/18/hurricanes-hit-the-poor-the-hardest/).

Brookings Institute. 2020. https://www.brookings.edu/blog/future-development/2020/05/05/the-unreal-dichotomy-in-covid-19-mortality-between-high-income-and-developing-countries/.

Craven, Pat. 2008. *Living with the Dominator: A Book About the Freedom Programme*. London: Freedom Publishing.

Criado Perez, Caroline. 2019. *Invisible Women: Exposing Data Bias in a World Designed for Men*. London: Chatto and Windus.

Crittenden, Pat. 2008. *Raising parents: Attachment, Parenting and Child Safety*. Cullompton, Devon: Willan.

Duffell, Nick, and Thurstine Bassett. 2016. *Trauma, Abandonment and Privilege*. London: Routledge.

Freud, Anna. 1966. *Normality and Pathology in Childhood: Assessments of Development*. London: Hogarth Press.

Hallegatte, Stephanie, A. Vogt-Schilb, J. Rozenberg, et al. 2020. From Poverty to Disaster and Back: a Review of the Literature. Economics of Disasters and Climate Change 4: 223–247. https://doi.org/10.1007/s41885-020-000 60-5

The Health Foundation. 2020. https://www.health.org.uk/news-and-comment/news/covid-19-now-is-the-time-to-redraw-the-uks-map-of-ine.

Joanna, Macrae, and Zwi Anthony. 1992. Food as an Instrument of War in Contemporary African Famines: A Review of the Evidence. *Disasters* 16: 299–321.

Lancet. 2020. https://www.thelancet.com/journals/lancet/article/PIIS0140-673 6(20)30893-X/fulltext.

Myers, Wayland. 1998. *Non-Violent Communication: The Basics as I Know and Use Them.* Encinitas, CA: Wayland Myers Books.

Orwell, George. 1969. *The Collected Essays, Journalism and Letters: An Age Like This, 1920–40*, vol. 1. London: Secker and Warburg.

Papali, Nina. 2019. A Meta-Analytic Review of the Efficacy of Psychological Treatments for Violent Offenders in Correctional and Forensic Mental Health Settings. *Clinical Psychology Science and Practice.* https://doi.org/10.1111/cpsp.12282.

Roy, Arundhati. 2020. Financial Times. 3/4/2020. https://www.ft.com/content/10d8f5e8-74eb-11ea-95fe-fcd274e920ca.

10

When Disaster Strikes

No single chapter can offer comprehensive guidance on how to respond when disaster strikes. The aim of this chapter is to summarize helpful strategies and provide signposts to existing resources. The perspective taken is how to respond when unwittingly caught up in a disaster that has hit one's community.

Naturally, in a disaster situation the first and highest priority is to preserve life, all other considerations are subordinate to that. The second is to protect and maintain the material circumstances that will make life in the present possible. Only when they are in place, can the third priority emerge which is the reconstruction work required to secure future life. Wrapped up in each of those priorities will be the emotional survival of people caught up in the disaster. And of extreme importance to understand is that material survival will be uppermost in survivor's minds, and all psychological considerations will be subordinate to that.

© The Author(s), under exclusive license to Springer Nature
Switzerland AG 2022
J. Woodcock, *Families and Individuals Living with Trauma*,
Palgrave Texts in Counselling and Psychotherapy,
https://doi.org/10.1007/978-3-030-79039-4_10

> **Learning Point**—Material survival will be uppermost in survivor's minds. Psychological considerations are secondary.

Evidence shows that until material life is possible few survivors have the capacity to engage in therapeutic and emotionally reparative work. However, family networks, neighborhood bonds and community relations need to be considered in the first phase of disaster planning because resilient communities emerge out of situations where relationships within the community have been strengthened by their consultation and involvement in disaster preparation and after-care. Usually unless civil society has been completely compromised by war or the scale of the disaster, there will be a framework for consultation and leadership within the community, and all emergency relief efforts will benefit from using that framework. Commonly there will be a disaster contingency plan, and authorities at state and local level will have practiced how this would be enacted, with key roles and responsibilities defined, and protocols in place to assess need and escalate responses as required. When this is not in place because of damage to civil society, non-governmental organizations such as the United Nations UN Disaster Assessment and Co-ordination (UNDAC), the Disasters Emergency Committee in the United Kingdom that co-ordinates the United Kingdom's international disaster relief response, and USAID in the United States provide these functions. Naturally in these situations, the necessity to involve actors in civil society is paramount. War can make this enormously difficult because the resources that the international community provides may become bargaining points between conflicting sides. The need for a supra-national response from key agencies like UNDAC is vital in these situations, and equal to this is the need for coherence between disaster relief efforts from different countries.

Psychological First Aid

Over the years of responding to therapeutic needs in disaster zones, an understanding has emerged of a basic toolkit required to respond effectively to the psychological needs of these situations. The protocol is widely accepted by national and international providers as the key to how to provide emergency psychological relief. The beauty of Psychological First Aid is that it is clear and simple, it has logical steps and a common sense framework that can be easily taught to people on the ground and this adds hugely to its effectiveness because frontline staff and local volunteers can be supported by more experienced workers, and people who need more intensive help are more easily identified within the framework. Psychological First Aid (NCTSN 2021) has eight core actions as follows:

1. Contact and Engagement: To respond to contacts initiated by survivors, or to initiate contact in a non-intrusive, compassionate, and helpful manner. To be led by their needs.
2. Safety and Comfort: To enhance and improve their immediate and ongoing safety, and to provide simple physical and emotional comfort.
3. Stabilization: To calm emotionally overwhelmed survivors and re-orient disoriented survivors, if this is required.
4. Information Gathering: To identify immediate needs and concerns, gather additional information, and tailor Psychological First Aid interventions.
5. Practical Assistance: To offer practical help to survivors in addressing their immediate needs and concerns.
6. Connection with Social Supports: To help establish contact with primary sources of support including family members, friends, and other persons and sources of support and help resources in the community.
7. Information on Coping: To provide information about stress reactions and coping to reduce distress and promote adaptive functioning.
8. Make Links with Collaborative Services: To link survivors with available services needed at the time or in the future.

These eight core actions enable psychological help to be rapidly dispersed and for it to be a seamless part of disaster provision because of the underlying philosophy that material needs and emotional well-being are intrinsic to each other, that survivors intrinsic means of resilience should be supported and that everything should be done to assist and promote existing social networks. These forms of help can also be easily explained to survivors, their families and adults and older children who are ready to assist including the simple forms of targeted help that are part of the package. Key elements in psychological first Aid are orientation and stabilization and they are described in these two boxes.

More Targeted Psychological Help

Psychological First Aid also allows for more targeted psychological help. Techniques for stabilization include advice on calming oneself through breathing and help with orientation, which are primarily ways of bringing survivors back in to the "here and now." These are similar to the interventions described in Chapter 7.

Exercise

Stabilization

1. Sit with your arms and legs uncrossed with your hands in your lap and your back as straight but relaxed as possible.
2. Breath in and out slowly and deeply. Count your breaths up to ten, and concentrate on your breath. When other thoughts and feelings come in, let them go and return to the breath.
3. Look around and notice five ordinary and non-distressing things you can see. Name each in turn and notice every detail of them with real intent. For instance, "Shoe, light blue with white stripes, and white laces, the laces half done up; tree, bare branches, two leaves moving in the breeze, buds forming."
4. Return to the breath and breath in deeply and slowly five more times.

---

5. Now name five non-distressing sound you can hear and describe them. For instance, "I hear a car on the road, it's sounds as if its driving slowly, I hear a woman talking, she's talking quite a lot and but slowly."
6. Return to the breath and breath in deeply and slowly five more times.
7. Now name five objects you can feel. For instance, "I feel the fabric of my jeans and my leg underneath, I feel my toes moving in my shoes."
8. Return to the breath: breath in and out slowly and deeply. Count your breaths up to ten, and concentrate on your breath. When other thoughts and feelings come in let them go.

Orientation also includes teaching survivors that intense feelings and reactions to disaster are very normal and common and that these do usually lessen over time but there are orientation and relaxation methods that can help.

Guidance

Orientation Advice

Intense emotions often come and go in waves.

Shocking experiences trigger strong and upsetting bodily reactions, such as strong alarm responses and startle reactions. These are completely normal.

Sometimes the best way to recover is to take time for a calming routine such as a walk, or breathing and muscle relaxation techniques.

Friends and family are important for support to calm down.

Children and adolescents when it's bad it's good to talk to your mum and dad to help you calm down.

Staying busy really helps. Offer to help if you can do practical things or organize a game with your friends.

Because bodily reactions are often strong after survival from disaster, it helps to teach some bodily relaxation skills. These are enormously helpful in disaster situations and anywhere where stress may be overwhelming.

Simple relaxation can include a breathing exercise, learning to breath deeply and slowly into the abdomen, placing the hands on the lower part of the tummy and making the hands rise and fall with each breath, and counting each breath in groups of ten and keeping that up for five minutes, or it can involve sitting or lying, closing the eyes and beginning with the feet taking turns to tense and then relax the muscles, and gradually moving up the body tensing and relaxing each group of muscles in turn. In the box, there is a slightly more elaborate relaxation that can work on one's own but is best led by someone else, this body scan relaxation can lead to a very deep sense of relaxation and self-healing.

Exercise

Body Scan Relaxation

1. Lie or sit somewhere comfortable
2. Close your eyes if you wish
3. Breathe in deeply and slowly, breath in so your tummy rises, let the breath go breathing out slowly and long. Scan your body, notice any areas that feel tight, uncomfortable, sore, attend to them, do they have a sound or vibration or particular sensation? Give them a color (different to your favorite color), imagine those areas wrapped in that color.
4. Breath in, imagine your breath is your favorite color, visualize the breath going right down into your left foot, filling your left foot with color, wiggle your toes and let your breath go, slowly.
5. As your warm colored breath encounters any area of discomfort imagine it filling it up and changing its color to your favorite color.
6. Breath in again, imagine your breath is your favorite color, visualize the breath going right down into your left leg below the knee, filling your left leg with color, feel its warmth filling you, let your breath go, slowly.
7. Breath in again, imagine your breath is your favorite color, visualize the breath going right down into your left leg from hip to toes, filling your left leg with color, feel your breath filling you and making your leg heavy and warm, let your breath go, slowly.

---

8. Work your way through each section of the body left leg, right leg, pelvis, lower abdomen, stomach, chest, shoulders, left hand, left arm below elbow, left arm, right arm, neck, back of head, face, forehead, crown of head.
9. Imagine body filled with the warm colored light that you have breathed in. All of you from head to toe filled with your favorite color, warm and heavy.
10. Relax and breathe gently, slowly.
11. Open your eyes and come back when you are ready.

Visualization

Visualizations are particularly powerful for enabling children to relax. The following visualization is good for any child over the age of 6–8 and it works just as well with older children and adults, and can be used with a whole group or a family.

Exercise

Visualization
1. Sit or lie somewhere comfortable and close your eyes if you can
2. Imagine yourself on a beach, you can hear the waves coming in very gently, the wind is warm and gentle against your face, the sun is warm.
3. Imagine getting up to your feet and walking by the sea, you feel the sea lapping over your feet.
4. In the water there are many shells, imagine the shells, reach down and pick one up.
5. Feel the shell in your hands, its shape and ridges, it inside and outside.
6. Collect another shell, place it in your other hand, and another, and another.

7. Fill your pocket with shells, hear them rattle a bit as they drop into your pocket.
8. Walk slowly away from the sea and up the beach.
9. Smooth out a piece of sand with your foot, slowly, feel the warm slightly wet sand under your feet as you smooth.
10. Take the shells and place them down one by one and write your name with the shells.
11. Use one last shell as a full stop.
12. Stand and look at your name, hear the sea behind you, the wind in the grass.
13. Pick up that last full-stop shell and put it in your pocket as a memento.
14. Feel it in your pocket as you walk up the beach.
15. Take a deep breath and open your eyes when you are ready.

An amazing resource for visualizations similar to that can be found in Mark Pearson's book *Emotional Healing and Self-Esteem* (2008). Mark's work was developed for use in schools in New South Wales, Australia to help children with relaxation, meditation, inner life skills, and the spillover from these practices is a natural deepening in classroom focus and concentration but they can be used anywhere, where events and feelings intrude and shake up the poise of the inner world.

Self-Help

Ways to help oneself, one's self definitions, and one's family and friends and community are hugely important in disasters (Eastmond, 2005). All the targeted help that agencies bring such as Psychological First Aid works on the principle that it will provide the impetus to enable the vast majority of survivors to help themselves and lend help to others. Self-help in disaster situations puts into action the basics of what is best about resilience.

Learning Point

Self Help and Resilience

- Being able to believe and make sense of what has happened.
- Having self-esteem—and this can emerge out of being able to act in ways that are protective of oneself and others.
- Being protective and loving and comforting toward oneself and others.
- Being able to achieve some things, however small, to make life more safe and more bearable.
- Learning new practical skills to aid survival.
- Learning and using emotional and relational skills that help others with survival—this may include helping others with stabilization and orientation.
- Using listening skills to help others survive emotionally —listening skills are paying attention using eye contact, giving small verbal "Uh huh, mmm-hmmm"), facial expressions (smiles, raised eyebrows, pursed lips) and physical responses (nodding your head) to show you are listening; giving small bits of feedback to show you have listened and have "got it"; not offering practical or emotional advice (that's quite hard to do) but just listening; and not judging.
- Working with others to achieve all of these gains.

Moving Beyond First Aid

Psychological First Aid is an excellent tool for bringing skills of emotional survival resilience to whole populations, these skills become embedded and that helps to unite and build resilient communities.

Guidance

What More In-depth Therapy Might Include if it can.

- Containment and validation of over-powering emotions
- Validation of experience in a non-intrusive survivor-led way
- Attention to bodily sensations

- Methods of relaxation
- The capacity to bring one into the present moment when dissociated
- The capacity to work with flashbacks and other intrusive effects
- An understanding of the nature of anxiety, its links to trauma and how to work with it
- An understanding of the roots of shame and guilt and reparation
- The ability to find meaning in events
- The capacity to provide a symbolic means to work through trauma through art, movement, play, music and drama.
- An understanding of how to work with the neurobiology of trauma.
- The capacity to work with dreams and nightmares.
- An understanding of the limits of help

These methods are also naturally good at identifying survivors who are too disturbed to be helped in these simple and effective ways, and they can be advised to seek the more intensive help that can be offered.

Therapists have engaged in the work of traumatic aftermath for years. After the Armenian earthquake of 1988 brief psychotherapy was offered in the back of a canvas-covered truck; art therapists Debra Kalmanovwitz and Bobbi Lloyd (1997) took the portable studio to the former Yugoslavia to work with survivors of political conflict, therapists worked in Sri Lanka in the aftermath of the tsunami, they have worked in communities and schools following mass shootings in the United States and Europe, and therapists are at work in tented refugee camps. The diversity of what can be offered may be confusing but there is some consensus about what should be included in what helps. Here is a list of what therapy might include. These approaches are covered in greater depth in previous chapters:

What We Can Do as Family and Friends

Consider all this together with the survivor and in your family/friendship circle, take turns to speak, listen, and reflect

Practice all the simple things set out in the boxes in this chapter.
Work to build community.
Draw on your own cultural wisdom.
Seek resources, help to guide and direct the help on offer.
NGOs should take great care to draw in the strengths of the community, to amplify the agency of those who have survived disaster, to ensure that practices are in place to prevent the exploitation of local staff and residents, to close the power differences between people who have survived disaster and those who come in to help, to create forums in which the actual experience of receiving psychosocial help are used openly to inform practice.

References

https://www.nctsn.org/sites/default/files/resources//pfa_field_operations_guide.pdf.

Eastmond, Marita. 2005. The Disorders of Displacement: Bosnian Refugees and the Reconstruction of Normality. In Managing uncertainty: Ethnographic studies of illness, risk and the struggle for control, ed. Vibeke Steffen, Richard Jenkins, and Hanne Jessen. Copenhagen: Museum Tusculanum Press.

Kalmanovwitz, Debra, and Bobbi Lloyd. 1997. *The Portable Studio Art Therapy and Political Conflict*. London: Health Education Authority.

Pearson, Mark. 2008. *Emotional Healing and Self-Esteem*. London: Jessica Kingsley.

11

Learning to Look After Ourselves

When asked how she looks after herself, a colleague of over thirty years who leads a team of therapists working with trauma said that she seeks stillness, stillness inside herself. She also realizes how reaching out to others and connecting, and moving beyond the deep interiority of being a psychotherapist is deeply important and nourishing. And being in contact with nature, knowing that she is deeply and intimately entwined in the natural world, that all its roots and branches and leaves, and rivers and streams, and hills and valleys and all those running, hunting, creeping, burrowing, swimming flying things are intimately and deeply part of her. This has been such an important aspect of her vitality since her childhood. These are the things that protect and sustain her, and yet she said, "I'm not awfully good at it, it's just a case of going on trying, being still, reaching out to others and being reached, and noticing how entwined with nature I am."

This is where this chapter starts, knowing that being with trauma has a deep effect on us, and learning to look after ourselves, and knowing always that this is a work in progress, there is no point of arrival, no mountain top where we arrive and are unassailable. The inevitability of

J. Woodcock, *Families and Individuals Living with Trauma*, Palgrave Texts in Counselling and Psychotherapy, https://doi.org/10.1007/978-3-030-79039-4_11

this work and of our lives is that the ground is always shifting beneath our feet, interests drop away even as horizons widen, new perspectives open up. Some years ago while considering work with refugees I wrote:

> We may seek a cure to the trauma that is alerted within us, but there is no cure to being touched by the human condition: there is no cure to being touched by compassion, and there is much to celebrate because this work can be done collectively and supportively in ways that maintain the most profound connections with our each other and the wider human family (Woodcock, 2014).

Hence caring for others is costly to ourselves and yet the rewards cannot be easily totted up like a balance sheet. Equally the costs are both sometimes dramatically obvious, but also subtle, elusive and difficult to pin down. We will delve into the costs and the reward, so they become recognizable.

Secondary Traumatic Distress

The most specific effect of caring for trauma is secondary traumatic stress, this is when the effects of trauma we have been working with or caring for in others begin to effect ourselves. Nowhere have these been more penetratingly and elegantly described as by Charles Figley in *Compassion Fatigue* (1995). Effects will vary between people so it is helpful to have a list of the components that make up the recognizable aspects of it. They are listed here as physical; cognitive, affecting the way we think and our overall capacity to think; emotional, effecting our feelings; behavioral, affecting the way we behave; existential, affecting our values and appreciation of life and our outlook; and interpersonal, the ways we interact with others. Nothing like all of these will affect everyone, but it is likely that if you are affected by one aspect from each of the categories that secondary traumatic stress is getting to you. If you have two or more, or twelve aspects from across the list, then you are pretty deeply affected and need help. If more than that you require immediate and careful attention.

If you are working regularly with trauma or have been caring for a loved one with trauma scan this list and see how many apply to you. Secondly, as a really important part of that self-scrutiny ask someone who knows you to run through the list and gently draw your attention to what they think fits (Table 11.1).

What to Do?

The question is what to do if you are hitting a dozen, or even less of these criteria? Begin with an honest appraisal. Also, because withdrawal is so often part of the picture, it is so important to do this exercise with someone else. Furthermore, if you are in a team or partnership and have noticed a team member or fellow carer somehow gradually withdrawing and having less to do with others, often in ways that seem entirely reasonable, until you stand back and look at it through this lens, then gently step forward and suggest they might do the appraisal. Run through the categories in turn and score yourself for any that fit. Don't be hard and fast about these labels, they are indicators and approximations, if you lean toward a criteria count it in the list. When you have finished consider what to do. There are two ways to take this—either remedial measures that allow you to look after yourself with greater care or some form of rest or withdrawal from the work.

> **Learning Point**—Work with trauma can bring a compelling blindness to one's own needs.

Remedial Measures

Remedial measures can include stepping back from the work for a while, such as by organizing a temporary rest from specific trauma work or a taking a holiday, or reducing your involvement with certain aspects

Table 11.1 The impact of trauma on carers—secondary traumatic stress

Physical	Cognitive	Emotional	Behavioral	Existential	Interpersonal
Shortness of breath	Diminished concentration	Anger	Irritability	Loss of purpose	Withdrawal
Panic	Forgetfulness	Fear	Impatience	Lack of self-satisfaction	Isolation
Nausea	Spaced out	Anxiety	Withdrawal	Hopelessness	Over-protective as parent
Palpitations	Disorientation Loss of self-worth	Nightmares Powerlessness	Sleep disturbance Changes in appetite	Ennui	
Aches and pains	Apathy	Numbness			Isolation from friends Intolerance
Dizziness	Rigid thinking Self-doubt Losing things	Guilt Sadness Depression Hypersensitivity Overwhelmed			
Jumpy Exaggerated startle response					
Frequent minor illnesses indicative of an impaired immunity	Over-preoccupied with trauma	Drained	Adoption of negative coping strategies, alcohol, prescription, and non-prescription drugs	Questions about the meaning of life	Withdrawal from emotional and sexual intimacy
		Shame			

of the work. If your involvement is with a loved one, this will almost certainly involve a discussion with them and ideas about how you step back, and if you need a complete rest who might need to step in while you take a break. Be honest with yourself, and with your colleagues and others involved. One of the outstanding things about work with trauma and secondary traumatic stress is that the compulsion to help can feel extraordinarily strong, and one can feel absolutely vital to the work or to the project. This is itself is quite a danger sign and is so common, and a compelling reason why people do not step back and seek help for themselves. These smaller remedial measures may not cut it, and a bigger step back may be necessary.

Learning Point

One of the outstanding things about work with trauma and secondary traumatic stress is that the compulsion to help can feel extraordinarily strong, and one can feel absolutely vital to the work or to the project. This in itself is quite a danger sign and is so common, and a compelling reason why people do not step back and seek help for themselves. So step back, seek help.

The next remedial measure is to accept help for yourself either through professional counselling or through a friend or colleague who commits to listening to you out, until you have the measure of what has been affecting you and have put in a course of contemplation and action to prevent you getting back to that place again. Of course there are no guarantee, and so as part of that it is vitally important to put in a review so once back in the fray you have a space you will drop into to check things out. This is vitally important because of the compelling blindness to one's own needs that work with trauma can bring about.

The next step to consider is whether one needs a complete break from the work, and this can be hard because the work is so compelling, often one's knowledge is very personal, seemingly indispensable and very specialist, and the relationships forged in trauma work are also very absorbing, deeply meaningful and even irresistible, so letting go of all of that is hard. Nevertheless, one has to give up the myth of indispensability, your stepping away frees up the possibility for someone else to step in with their unique skills, and if done in a timely and well-considered manner, you can act as an advisor or mentor as they find their feet.

Daily and Weekly Self-Care

Next, we need to consider daily and weekly self-care, the sorts of things we can do to hold us from falling too deeply into forgetfulness of our needs. The list of things proposed by my friend and colleague at the start of the chapter is a good starting point: seeking stillness within; reaching out to others, and allowing oneself to be reached, and immersion in nature. Nature has a compellingly restorative feel because of the cycle of the seasons. We experience winter stripping leaves from the trees and plants, and returning the land to bare earth, and driving birds and animals into sleep and migration. And every spring there is renewal, the breaking forth of buds and the arrival of migrants. This teaches us that renewal is perennial and we can be part of it. Because trauma exerts such a toll on our physical selves, being out in nature is a powerful remedy. Walking, running, swimming and other physical exercise allow our bodies to consume re-regulate adrenaline and its by-product of cortisol, which when released in excess in response to chronic stress can remain elevated and lead to high blood pressure, anxiety, sleep problems, weight gain, and poor memory and concentration.

Learning Point

Cortisol is released to allow the liver to release glucose stores for fight and flight; under repeated or chronic stress these remain elevated and can dysregulation of the Hypothalamus-Pituitary-Axis (HPA) or stress response system and lead to raised blood pressure, heart disease, sleep problems, weight gain, depression, anxiety, and poor memory and concentration.

The fact that these stress chemicals and stress responses have such a dramatic effect on the body highlights why *daily* physical activity is such an antidote to stress, and why finding silence within, quieting oneself, breathing deeply, stretching, and activities like yoga are so good at countering secondary traumatic stress.

Guidance

The key to each of these activities is that they have both an active engaging component and a reflective component. Anyone who has ever run knows that it involves not only physical effort but also delivers a wonderful, deeply reflective state of mind; people who do yoga are aware that it demands physical effort and also commands phases of active attention and letting go; reading requires the almost passive following of a narrative, along with an actively engaged mind that makes sense of what unfolds; connecting to family and friends also requires that we are reciprocal, and meditation may seem like a place where we are alone and passive but it almost certainly brings us into a pace wherein the quiet we are visited by thoughts, and feelings and sensations, they arrive, we pay them brief focused attention, we may even interrogate them, and then we let them go (Table 11.2).

Table 11.2 Activities that counter stress

Daily physical activity	Relaxation	Connecting	Finding silence
Walking	Yoga	Family	Meditation
Running	Music	Friends	Being in Nature
Swimming	Stretching	Colleagues	Walking
Cycling	Reading	Supervision	
Gardening	Arts and	Community	
Fitness		Eating well	

> **Learning Point**
>
> Secondary traumatic stress involves overwhelm and hopelessness and helplessness on one side and on the other side dissociation, forgetfulness, distraction, anxiety, and denial. The best antidote to that stress are activities that have an active engaging component that engages with the physical effects and a reflective component. Hard physical activity reabsorbs cortisol; reflection strengthens our capacity to mentalise and to be metacognitive.

The Hidden Effects of Stress

We imagine that therapists are fairly conscious folk, after all the training demands that they receive therapy, practice reflection with colleagues, keep journals of their inner lives, and most continue this inner work diligently through their working lives. We might imagine because of this they would clock the effects of stress on themselves but I have to say they aren't particularly good at it. My doctoral research (2006) set out to understand how secondary traumatic stress affected psychotherapists and what it revealed was that they were effected in ways of which they were conscious such as episodes of low mood, anxiety, irritability, poor concentration, sometimes a sense of hopelessness in the face of the overwhelming nature of the work but they were also affected even more deeply and persistently in ways of which they were barely conscious.

There are at least three reasons why the barely conscious effects of secondary trauma are held at bay, and kept out of mind. The first and most simple is because it's hard and troubling to think about, perhaps even more deeply so when our drive is toward helping others in a way that puts our own needs aside, sometimes because we have fantasies about being invulnerable, sometimes because we are inexperienced and don't expect the work to get to us like it inevitably will. The second is because we have an inner compulsion to do the work that has emerged out of our own past trauma, great or small, and it's hard to distinguish the affects of our own stuff from the stuff of work, so anxiety, flashes of fear, overwhelm, and being a bit dissociated feel like familiar territory. In addition, the inner compulsion to heal others as a way of attending to our own wounds is often driven by powerfully unconscious forces. To take an analogy from astro-physics, of which I know nothing, it is as if we can be aware of the event horizon, the fact that the black hole is there, but beyond that point no light, and in the case of unconscious mental forces, no understanding or insight escapes. The third is because we have inklings that the work is hurting us but no one to confirm our suspicions because there aren't the forums where this is thought about. In work this may be because the pace of work is so frantic, often because work with people is prioritized over therapist's needs, and this is right up to a point, as long as space is given in a thoughtful and well-punctuated way to raising consciousness about these issues so they can be addressed in ways that are most fitting to individuals and the institutions where they work, and for family members caught up in caring for traumatized loved ones, space given to considering how it will effect them alongside strategies for working with one's loved ones.

Pain and Memory

Several years ago I gave a talk to the therapists and medical staff at a human rights organization in London where I had worked much of whose work is with people traumatized. The purpose was to share the findings of my research study to which many of them had generously contributed. It can be difficult to raise these issues, even with colleagues where there is deep mutual respect because one lifts the lid on quite how damaging the work can be, and one wishes to be measured and respectful of colleague's vulnerabilities and sensitivities, and supportive of morale and of the work. The message, "This work is damaging you" can be hard to hear. It was an interesting evening. Afterward a senior psychotherapist spoke to me about their deeply worrying experience of being referred to a leading London hospital for neurological diseases because of early signs of memory loss. However, after extensive tests, nothing had been found. They were deeply grateful for an explanation for their unexplained memory loss because my research had shown that one of the effects of work with trauma can be distinct effects of confusion and memory impairment. As far as can be determined, these are not structural changes but psychological effects, forms of dissociation where the capacity to concentrate and remember are compromised. What is so fascinating is that memory becomes unreliable, as if one is viewing a distant scene through clouds, sometimes the view is quite distinct, sometimes as if lost in the fog. Most interestingly this carries through from the work itself through to annoying memory impairments in one's personal life. However, once stress is lowered good memory returns.

Learning Point—One needs to gently and supportively enquire how things are going in colleagues personal life, this is often where the dark shadows from work are cast.

It is not only memory impairment that carries through into life at home but also irritability, raised anxiety, lowered mood, and very often the people we live with suffer the ill consequences of these effects because we are less guarded with them. We show our best sides to our colleagues and clients or patients, those at home get licked by our moods. This compartmentalization is part of trauma and secondary trauma and is a good reason why in offering support and supervision, one needs to gently and supportively enquire how things are going in colleague's personal life, this is often where the dark shadows from work are cast.

How We Are Affected

The following is a list of the ways we are affected by the work. It is compiled in three columns, the obvious effects at the top and the less obvious and hidden effects below; how to notice, and what to do. The is a summary and far from comprehensive about how to spot things and what to do but it is an indicator of what to look for, and how to respond (Table 11.3).

Table 11.3   Guidance—secondary traumatic effects

	How to notice	What to do
Anxiety	Feel worried a lot of the time	Reflective talking/exercise
Low mood	Feel life is less enjoyable	Reflective talking/exercise
Intrusive ideas	Difficult thoughts pop into one's mind	Acknowledge/come into the present
Irritability	Feel more easily annoyed	Acknowledge/breathing
Anger	Feel angry more often	Acknowledge/ reflective talking/exercise/breathing
Preoccupied	Get lost in thought	Acknowledge/come into the present
Sadness	Sad feelings	Grieve what can't be changed/work for what can be changed/teach yourself and others the difference
Hidden anxiety	Distracted by worries that one tries to deny: use hospital anxiety and depression scale	Unearth and acknowledge anxieties; examine how relaxed is breathing, heart rate; use breathing, exercise
Depression	Low energy, low confidence, irritable, angry, sad; use hospital anxiety and depression scale	Reflective talking/exercise
Nightmares	Wake frightened at night	Keep a dream journal; practice being a conscious dreamer
Memory issues	Forget key things one ordinarily remembers	Step back from the work; take enough time out to come back into your own mind
Poor concentration	Easily distracted/lose train of thought/tasks take longer	Step back from the work; take enough time out to come back into your own mind
Dissociated	Spaced out	Meditation/breathing exercises; come into the present; find ways to anchor oneself in the present
Jumpy	Easily startled/Jumpy	Relaxation; breathing; meditation; rest

(continued)

Table 11.3 (continued)

	How to notice	What to do
Withdrawn	Isolation at work/not reaching out to friends or loved ones	

Forms of Self-Protection

There are forms of self-protection that therapists slip into without neces-sarily realizing it. Quite a number of those I questioned said they no longer followed the news, or listened to the radio or watched the tele-vision, or watched films and movies if there was anything disturbing or violent about them. Some found they stopped reading novels because the effort of attending to the inner world of others, which novels convey, was no longer rewarding and nourishing, it was as if their inner world was over-stuffed with trauma. Others continued to read but turned away from novels and biographies where people came to harm; they said they couldn't bear people they had made an emotional relationship with coming to harm.

Compartmentalization

It is common in trauma for experience to be compartmentalized, this helps us to deal with things that would otherwise overwhelm us. It is a form of splitting that brings to the fore a coping response and buries the feelings. Therapists do this too as a way of coping, there's them at work strong, organized, mostly cheerful and urbane (as far as everyone can see), and there's them at home, possibly miserable, distracted, irritable, more angry than they'd like to be, listless, tired, sleeping poorly, anxious, and jumpy. Because of this it is important to ask therapists how they are in their personal life, and as honestly as your relationship permits to wonder and ask the systemic circular question, how do key members of their close emotional network experience them? To do this with respect, and compassion and care, so as to invite a self-reflexive take on how they are, even if it's not answered, to set the hare of heuristic enquiry running, as it were.

Learning Point

Secondary trauma interferes with our capacity to be fully reflective, it diminishes preoccupies and concentration, and flattens our ability to take a third, reflexive position, looking in on ourselves. When someone is secondarily traumatized their capacity to be metacognitive is diminished.

It is compartmentalization also that hides some of the effects of doing the work from therapists themselves, although these are hiding in plain sight. Therapists, and people supporting loved ones, find that the way they absorb stress often mirrors the traumatized people they are setting out to help, as the list above shows, but there's a cognitive trick we play on ourselves, we're helping *them* so *we* can't suffer from these same things, can we? The truth is we do but compartmentalization into them and us protects us from easily seeing how we are affected. Instead, certain levels of stress are accepted as part of the job. Furthermore, secondary trauma interferes with our capacity to be fully reflective, it diminishes preoccupies and concentration, and flattens our ability to take a third, reflexive position, looking in on ourselves. As we saw in earlier chapters when someone is traumatized their capacity to be metacognitive is diminished. The dilemma is how to assess whether stress has become unbearably toxic. Here are some key questions:

Questions to Subjectively Determine if Stress Is at Breaking Point

1. Does taking a complete break from the work allow you to get back into your own mind?
2. Are you more persistently anxious than feels good for your well-being?

3. Are the negative emotions generated by the work jeopardizing your personal relations?
4. Do poor memory and concentration interfere with the quality of your life and work?
5. Is your low mood more persistent than feels good to you?
6. Are you feeling hopeless more than you would wish?
7. Are intrusive thoughts present more than you would wish?
8. Is your sleep persistently affected?
9. Can you switch off from work completely?
10. Do support and supervision help enough?
11. Does taking a complete break from the work allow you to get back into your own mind?
12. Have you given yourself free permission to leave if you need, and can you?

When these questions are asked we won't arrive at an objective opinion, everyone will have a different matrix of resilience, but it can help to arrive at a subjective assessment of how big a break does one need to get back into one's own mind; what changes can be put in place to make the situation more manageable; what is the nature of support they will find most useful, and can it be found?

Compassion Fatigue and Secondary Traumatic Stress

One of the costs of caring is compassion fatigue as detailed in great depth by Charles Figley and colleagues (1995). Compassion fatigue is a danger above and beyond the finer detail of secondary traumatic stress. It is a blanket term to describe a range of effects that anyone caring for others over a length of time may experience, and all carers are vulnerable to it. It is cognitively expensive to look after others who are traumatized, the work is complex, affecting and vital to human survival, and because of that, it is very compelling. Simple signs of compassion fatigue are that we are worn out, we lose the sense we had of infinite creative energy, our capacity to ask complex questions reduces and we start to see things in a narrower, almost predictable way, our curiosity becomes more blunt, we may be invaded by helplessness and hopelessness. These are very acute signs of compassion fatigue that indicate that we need to have an appraisal of our coping. The questions that are relevant here are:

1. How are you feeling?
2. Does your decision-making feel good?
3. Do your energy levels feel equal to the task?
4. Do you feel adequately supported?
5. Does your work feel valued?

If *any* of these are answered negatively a fast supportive response is required.

Looking After Ourselves When It's a Family Who Is Traumatized

When we are caring for family members who are traumatized, everything in this chapter should be food for thought and yet we need to give ourselves permission to care for ourselves. We know this can be especially difficult because we know our loved one and their needs like no one else. Even so, there is a compelling argument for giving ourselves space because the alternative can be collapse. The five questions above about compassion fatigue are very important, and the twelve questions to determine whether stress is at breaking point are equally important. Answering these means being up-front about what bothers us about being a carer, wrestling with our loyalty to ourselves, other family members and our traumatized loved one; admitting to ourselves what feels unbearable and negotiating the space required to come back into your own mind. This can be as simple as a regular day away when someone else steps in and regular time to put other relationships first and give them priority. Reaching out to others who can help, and briefing them as honesty as you can about what is most supportive to you; taking time to put in place measures that support your well-being, physical exercise, relaxation, breathing, and reflection.

> **Guidance**—Step back from work as a carer. Take enough time out to come back into your own mind.

Finally, there is a triad of positions to consider in this work of looking after ourselves, the first is the inevitability of being touched by the suffering of others, and this is deeply felt when it is our loved ones who are suffering. Another position in the triad is the equally human need to look after ourselves. There is a tension between these two places that needs to be held for the sake of our emotional survival, and some people resist the idea that they should look after themselves when immersed in caring for others. The third position one can take is gaze aversion, which is the act, sometimes unconscious, of looking the other way: we do that in order to protect ourselves. The work of this chapter has been how to properly understand and hold the tension between those three places. In my opinion, the healthiest position is one that encapsulates all three, care for others, that contains space to care for ourselves; the capacity to consider and work with the suffering of others, and the self-realization and self-possession to be able to step away and look after ourselves. Only when we are nourished can we nourish others. Years ago, an African woman who was in a desperate situation, separated from her children and with an uncertain future in exile said to me, "My situation is completely wretched but it is so important to me that you are in good heart. I want that for you so you can care for me, and I want it for you as a symbol of what I will one day be restored to myself." This work touches and changes us deeply, it causes deep existential changes whereby material needs become less important, and instead relationships and the deeper meaning of life shine forth. It is that place that encapsulates those three positions outlined above, a place of deep and nourishing reflection, and a lived three-cornered connection with our human family where we see, and reach out and act, and are nourished by a web of connections.

What We Can Do as Family and Friends

Consider All This Together with the Survivor and in Your Family/Friendship Circle, Take Turns to Speak, Listen, and Reflect

Consider how can I be compassionate to yourself, and ask how can we be compassionate to ourselves?

Work out how to step back, take time out

Consider how do we, and how do I find support?

Work out how I show and admit vulnerability?

Run through the questions in the chapter above to subjectively see if your stress is at breaking point, ask how are you doing; invite someone to be your breaking point support mentor, and you be theirs

Enjoy nature

Take exercise, and find time for relaxation, connecting, silence

References

Figley, Charles, ed. 1995. *Compassion Fatigue: Coping with Secondary Traumatic Stress Disorder in Those Who Treat the Traumatized*. Levittown, PA: Brunner/Mazel.

Woodcock, Jeremy. 2014. My Veins Don't End in Me: On Surviving Work with Survivors. Paper Given at the 19:e Nordiska konferesen forbehandlare som arbiter med traumatiserade flyktingar, Goteborg, 22–23 maj 2014.

12

Mainly Theory

This chapter takes a deeper dive into the theories that underpinned the thinking in previous chapters and also sets out to widen the scope of ideas presented in the book. It is written mainly for therapists but as far as possible, the ideas are made accessible for the general reader.

Trauma theory has burgeoned over recent years with two powerful trends clearly at work in the psychological domain, namely attachment theory and neurobiology, which are themselves also increasingly integrated. Whereas twenty years ago it was possible to discuss attachment theory as a coherent set of ideas, without much reference to neurobiology that is next to impossible now. An increasingly accurate understanding of interactions of brain and body has emerged in neuroscience that deeply informs how attachment, which always had deeply emotional-physiological roots, is understood. However, trauma is far too complex a phenomena to be entirely captured within psychological frameworks and for us to properly appreciate its depths, we need to turn to culture and sociology, history, literature, politics, and power, but let's begin with psychology.

© The Author(s), under exclusive license to Springer Nature
Switzerland AG 2022
J. Woodcock, *Families and Individuals Living with Trauma*,
Palgrave Texts in Counselling and Psychotherapy,
https://doi.org/10.1007/978-3-030-79039-4_12

My own professional pathway through this began working as a psychotherapist with survivors of torture at a human rights organization in London, it is also right to acknowledge prior experience of personal trauma while "in care" as a child. One of the fascinating things about trauma is how the personal and professional jostle for attention, how the emotional energy from one domain of experience flows into the other, and how good trauma is at infiltrating, how by definition at the very heart of the experience it lacks containment, and spills over messily. Everyone working with trauma will have been touched by its power to be no respecter of boundaries, to enter by the back door, and this makes it a fascinating and dangerous teacher.

Trauma is woven through the very historical fabric of psychotherapy, and like a thread in a complex tapestry, it appears and disappears, sometimes so successfully that entering the world of trauma, one has the experience of inventing the work anew, only to discover one's forbears were exactly there, struggling with its newness, its protean capacity to decorate human experience with new miseries. Are we the same creatures as the French fusilier at the siege of Rouen who found himself gazing into the terrified eyes of his companion, astonished as he died without a visible mark upon his body? Was this in 1592 a manifestation of traumatic terror that killed him? We will never know, and even if the physical experience of what happened to that fusilier may be similar to experiences in recent wars, arguably the cultural conditions make it entirely different. What brings us to this is that there is undoubtedly a huge tension in this work of how perception shapes and makes experience. Psychology by trying to place itself at the center of experience, even in the cerebral cortex itself, might believe it has found the indivisible quantum but this itself is an illusion because we continually precede ourselves, and we are more shaped by expectation and cultural freight than we can perhaps imagine. This is the shifting context that shapes all this work and from where we must begin as we consider the presence of the body in trauma.

The Presence and Absence of the Body in Psychotherapy

The fault line that runs through trauma theory is the presence of the body, and this begins with the Freudians. Trained as a neurologist, Freud was deeply attentive to the body, influenced by colleagues Jean-Martin Charcot and Pierre Janet, he rigorously pursued the puzzle as to how people who were otherwise fit and healthy seemed compelled into states of physical helplessness. What emerged in the talking cure as he turned away from hypnosis, was the complex logic that the unconscious plays in trauma. However, although trauma circulates through these early discoveries, it holds no organizing centrality. Freud has been criticized for turning his attention away from a direct knowledge of bodily experiences of the actual trauma that overwhelmed and entrapped his patients in the deeply repressed norms of early twentieth-century European culture, so their only medium of communication were forms of hysteria. As a result the theoretical complexity of psychoanalysis as it emerged mirrors the body in trauma, but reflects knowledge of it elsewhere rather than paying it direct attention. It could be said rather crudely that the troubles of the body were reflected and transposed into a theory of mind (Jones 1961; Gay 1988). The body did retain its presence but in transmuted form, present as libido, lurking in the erotic transference, appearing and disappearing as psychosomatic medicine in different cultural contexts but never getting real traction (Kurzweil 1989). In a sense, Freud and the Freudians are not to blame for this because the whole weight of the Western tradition drives us in the direction of a radical split between body and mind. This tendency has played its way through psychotherapy thinking up until the present day, while the actual experience of trauma has been to insist on the primacy of the body.

Shell Shock and Work in Groups

This split between mind and body compellingly reveals itself in the stories of shell shock from the First World War, where for instance embodied experiences of terror were responded to with electrical treatment of the body, however it can be argued that the intention was not to fix the body but to restore the mind. Furthermore, the apparent barbarism of these physical treatments was largely rejected in favor of versions of the talking cure (Shephard 2000). This trend continued in the Second World War, in the hands of sophisticated practitioners like the psychiatrist and psychoanalyst Wilfrid Bion, who writes compellingly in his memoir of his own experiences on the Western Front in the First World War in France as a tank commander (Bion 1982). His contributions to psychoanalysis were outstanding, his work with traumatized soldiers all too brief. Working as an army psychiatrist, he organized men surviving shell shock into groups to process the consequences of their experience but because he believed rank should be dissolved for the purposes of the therapeutic work, conflict emerged with the military authorities that cut his work short (Bléandonu 1994). Emerging from this work as a war psychiatrist, Bion's singular contribution to trauma work was to map out how anxiety compelled certain sets of behaviors in groups. These ideas later fed into Family Therapy, through Robyn Skynner (1987a), who understood the ways that groups behave as families and conversely how families behave as groups. What Bion conjectures is that we fear real intimacy in groups, and this fear creates vulnerability that compels three different defensive group responses. One is *fight or flight* in which the therapeutic group gets lost in fights among itself, or into real and symbolic fights with figures or wider organizations outside. Or it goes into flight, indulging in flights of fancy and fantasy, taking its mind anywhere but on the focus of what the central task of the group is, which is to relate openly and honestly and intimately with each other. The second compulsion that the group engages in order to avoid intimacy is *pairing*. This manifests in various ways, one may be a paring between a couple in the group that takes hold of everyone with utter fascination, playing out with frissons of emotional, intellectual, or sexual energy. But this is not real intimacy, it has the character of an electrifying flirtation. Pairing can play out in more mundane ways, such as when a member of the group makes an affiliation with the group leader, which becomes a defensive norm that prevents other intimate affiliations from emerging. A third compelling response is *dependence*, where typically group members experience themselves as without personal autonomy and absolutely dependent on the group leader, or on the organization in which the group is set. Bion conjectured that when these compulsions are worked through, the group can emerge into a mature form where it may be described as a *work group*, in which members relate to each other honestly and with intimacy, conflicts are acknowledged and explored, vulnerability is easy revealed, affiliations are genuine and fluid and there is a high degree of personal autonomy.

When we relate these ideas to trauma, it can perhaps be seen how valuable group work can be in working through traumatic experience. Trauma can deeply interfere with our capacity for intimacy, affiliation and autonomy. Also, fight and flight, dependence, and pairing with just one other in whom we trust absolutely are common features of the traumatic response, the long work of groups is brilliant at working through these manifestations of trauma. In addition, groups allow for the powerful identifications between survivors to work in a very positive way. For instance, the sense of alienation that survivor's experience, whereby they believe no one ordinary can conceive or understand what they have endured is overcome in groups where everyone shares this common bond. Slow though it may be to reveal itself, over time as trust and intimacy develop, the doing and undoing of identification becomes a powerful agent of change. To be understood by others so deeply through shared identification is incredibly affirming that the inner world of trauma, can actually be understood and shared. The task that follows this is that the group leader has to open up the intense intimacy and identification of the group to examination, so idealization can be worked through and similar affiliations can be made outside the group. The danger otherwise is that what develops is an almost holy truth that the group is the sole unique place where one can be understood. This is good for part of the process of healing but it can take on the character of the basic assumptions, where identification becomes a powerful form of pairing, or a form of flight from intimacy in the world outside, or a form of dependency on the group as the sole repository of our deeper trust (Woodcock 1997, 2001).

Fear of Intimacy and Projective Identification

To link back to absence of the body in trauma, what emerged in the second wave of psychoanalytic work of which Bion was part, was that the body manifested mostly not as a thing-in-itself but in the fear of intimacy. Ideas focused on the terror of intimacy, the fear of annihilation in the mental life of the other, the jostling of the libidinal oedipal currents, and other powerful manifestations of our psychic life that threaten to engulf and crush the delicate emergent mind. In that same context, projective identification became a powerful tool that emerged out of the Kleinian world. This pursued the notion that the patient projects into the psychotherapist their undigested, unthinkable experience, and that the job of the therapist is to make this conscious to themselves, and then as the patient develops and can bear it, to feed this knowledge back to them. In this process, the body is very much present, gut instinct is at work, and horrors transmitted into the therapist are experienced as bodily sensations, but the work is to render all into thought. It is thought that can be resolved out of this, seemingly, not bodily experience. It is clarity of thought that liberates, not physical experience. Projective identification is undoubtedly an incredibly valuable resource when working with trauma. It can feel as if one is being assaulted from within, and sorting out what belongs to one's own experience and what comes into one from the survivor is an extremely useful exercise that frees up the therapist to work with what is going on. However, it is important not only to bear this assault and feed it back when the survivor might be ready as ideas, hypotheses, and interpretations but to delve in and investigate the actual felt experience, as a bodily experience—in other words, beginning with can it be felt *bodily* as much as can it be known *intellectually*. However, this commentary is not intended to play down the incredible power of words, the wonderful capacity of psychotherapy to bring things into mind, to make what was hidden known, to render experience into thought Furthermore, there is the opportunity that trauma brings, dreadful though it is, to deliver us into a process of psychotherapy that is profound, and which will venture far beyond the original territory of trauma that propelled us here.

The Body as Container

Naturally in this partial account of the absence of the body in psychotherapy there are happy exceptions. For instance, there is Esther Bick's wonderful account of the experience of the skin in early object relations (1988), where the baby's early experience is deeply held in mind, and transforms into thinking about the containment of the therapeutic setting as a metaphor for the skin, literally holding the experience together. However, the tendency for actual bodily experience to be resolved away into ways of thinking is still powerfully present. There is also the powerful visceral experience of love and hate deeply present in the psychoanalytic canon, and discussion of its manifestations often takes up the full scope of the feeling realm, and the puzzle of how feeling states emerge from instinct. In his chapter on love and hate and the primal scene, Martin Stanton (2002) describes how the experiential registers, that is language and experience, "even though they enmesh and intertwine in everyday life.... are not readily inter-translatable." The question still lurks, however, if language and bodily experience intertwine how do we engage with bodily experience, not merely as thought but in actuality. Many clues to this are provided within Dinora Pines's *A Woman's Unconscious Use of Her Body* (1994), in her writing there is a powerfully constant tidal pull between body, its instincts and experience as deeply understood within the revealing canon of her theoretical position.

Containment and Validation

Containment and validation and bearing witness are essential to this work and Dick Blackwell writes about these themes with delicacy in

"Holding, containing and bearing witness" (1997). He takes up the sometimes overwhelming, and unhelpful impulse toward helpfulness, in distinction to the hard work of bearing witness to massive inner pain. Susan Levy (2004) also discusses how following trauma, the profound feelings of hate that sometimes emerge, create the need for containment and validation. Massive loss often entails massive guilt, and the other pole of this state of mind, which is the belief often presented by survivors that they must be really hated to have suffered so much. What is required in this situation is love and containment by the therapist, and the working through to a deep validation of experience. This validation has several elements—key among them the exploration and acknowledgment of *actual* experience, felt in all its dimensions, in the body, in the mind. Secondly, the experience as a metaphor, in what cannot be felt in a conscious way or thought about at first but can gently be brought to the surface over time. Thirdly, the experience as felt emotionally, being full of guilt, or shame, even feeling hated by life itself. For instance, an Ethiopian man who crawled away from a disaster on his hands and knees, had legs that later gave way constantly at the knees. He began to see where this weakness originated but even though validated quite simply, it did us no good in our work together. It was when we got hold of the metaphors of how utterly infantile he felt, weakened, overlooked, guilty because unable to help others, hated and feeling hatred because abandoned, and how this resonated with a great deal of his original early experience, and able to feel attention and love in the therapeutic relationship, and finally to offer love back to himself that he was able to literally get back on his feet again.

Shame

Shame is another emotion frequently felt in trauma. Again it can have its origins in things done or not done. Babette Rothschild refers helpfully to amygdala, which triggers the flow of adrenaline that compels us to fight or run or hide (2010) even before thought arrives. When we give instinctive priority to our bodily survival over others, how can we be blamed for that which we do instinctively? However, shame lodges so deeply perhaps not simply because it is triggered by such a primitive aspect of our functioning, but also because in our development, it merges with the helplessness of our bodies, our dependence on the love and pleasure or disgust of those who attend to our basic bodily functions. Shame brings us into contact with all of that, and as often is the case with trauma, the way out of the clinging thicket of its experience is to take up not only the actual experience in all its dimensions but the shadows it throws onto our early development. In this respect, traumatic experience can be a tremendous, if horrible opportunity, to work through early experience. Furthermore, because much of that is preverbal working with unthought bodily experienced material, with projection, and the myths, and dreams and stories of our beginnings is rich and vital part of the work. An Ethiopian man, adopted by his uncle, proud of his family and yet shamed not to be raised by his poor parents bumped up against all these contending themes as we worked together.

Attachment Theory

Cutting across all the psychotherapies, causing dissension and alarm in psychoanalytic circles, from where its outstanding practitioner sprang, was John Bowlby. It is astonishing to think that his work remains controversial to them, even now. Perhaps less so when one considers that what he bumped against was real experience when they were deeply wedded to the notion of phantasy. What Bowlby's work with Mary Ainsworth and the strange situation established was an ethological view of child development tempered with the growth of mind, whereby it is our internal working model of self and relationships, developed out of actual experience, both bodily and mental, that guides us in the conduct of our key relationships. Little will be added here, other than a deep acknowledgment of how vital to an understanding of trauma is this groundbreaking work in the developmental field.

What then proceeds out of Bowlby, if not always in straightforward ways, are many other important developments that are vital to work with trauma. The list should include Peter Fonagy's continued work on metallization and affect regulation (2002). Here the links between actual relational experience and the capacity for affect regulation and reflective function are themes that are deeply informative of work with trauma. Much of what has been covered in this book works with that edge where bodily experience is acknowledged, supported, contained, brought into language, and metamorphosed. It is as if at this moment, a great deal of work in this area coincides with these ideas, although I would not wish to do any a disservice by over identifying each with the other. What comes into mind however is the work of Daniel Seigal bringing child development, attachment, neurobiology, and mindfulness together; Felicity de Zulueta writing about human violence as a preventable disease (2004) and the profound and compelling links she makes between pain as a bodily and psychic experience and the intergenerational transmission of trauma (1993).

Vietnam War Veterans

War has always pushed medical and psychological studies forward and this is so very true of the Vietnam War that challenged America for so many generations. Emerging out of work with veterans Bessel Van Der Kolk brings together a profound understanding of the neurobiology of trauma that has made use of an understanding of the neurological workings of early attachment, and the neurobiology of traumatic adult experience (1987). His *The Body Keeps the Score* (2015) has to be a starting point for anyone venturing to understand or work with trauma. Here, as the title suggests, the body and its experiences are both known, and allowed into thought, and allowed to be known through finely graduated attention to subjective sensations and the therapist's attention to outward bodily signs. What is so fine about this book is how easily and well it communicates key facts to the general reader.

The work of Judith Lewis Herman also stands out as *the* place where one should start reading about trauma. Her work teases apart the similarity and differences between complex developmental trauma and later single event traumas, and she speaks from an impassioned place of discovery. Key among Lewis Herman's ideas is the power of forgetting, not just as a personal experience but as a set of interacting social and political events. Her work, although long before, is a precursor that enables us to understand the power of the *Me Too* movement to unearth in powerfully debated terms why the voices of survivors are so readily pushed underground, unless we have courage to join up, speak up, and face down oppression. Trauma silences and alienates us from ourselves, from others, and from our own lived experience and in the face of this, the need to connect is a vital theme that runs through her writing. Working with teams that work with trauma, sometimes the politics of survivors and the clinic coincide in such a way as to push colleagues into the margins. These are the moments to catch, reflect, and reach out to those with whom we work: the work is hard enough.

Unclaimed Experience

Writing powerfully about unclaimed experience is Cathy Caruth from within the field of literature. In an edited collection by Caruth (1995) Dori Laub, speaks to the sense in survivors of "being in a "secret order" that is sworn to silence (Laub 1995). The requirement therefore is for psychotherapist to be witness, and for something to be created relationally where "the listener is established in the mind" of the survivor. Here is psychoanalysis deeply understanding the silencing, the splitting freight of trauma, of experience disappeared from the mind because it is not only too terrifying to recall but because so many cultural injunctions stand in the way of its expression. This is work that Dori Laub and Nanette Auerhahn gave voice to in *Knowing and Not Knowing massive Psychic Trauma* (1993), where conscious the levels at which traumatic experience can be known are elegantly traced from the unconscious, through the body and into survival that compels us into living out life themes that have traumatic origins. Among our colleagues and survivors working in the field, one knows this compulsion, and the question, how to rest with it is never simple. Caruth has pressed on with her work interviewing practitioners and capturing the dislocated, fragmentary and bizarre ways that trauma surfaces and her work's vitality lies in the way it transcends categories of knowledge just as trauma does itself.

EMDR

Within the strict observance of its therapeutic protocols, Eye Movement Desensitization and Reprocessing (EMDR) is a long way from the free association out of which literature emerges, and yet it seems there is in some ways an unbroken arc between Freud's work with hypnosis and EMDR. It seems to me to be much like a sub-hypnotic technique, although one where the protocol holds the survivor in a zone akin to the window of tolerance. The instruction is to look in on one's experience as if at a distance, as if looking out from the window of a passing train. Very often though the survivor gets sucked into the bodily experience of the narrative, and the skill of the practitioner is to hold that edge between a new experience where the trauma is reprocessed, and one where the survivor may be re-traumatized. It is the gap between these outcomes that no doubt has lent itself to EMDR trainings being extended. My own practice has been to use it within the confines of an already established therapeutic relationship where safety is implicit, and where the protocols within the technique that makes safety explicit is temporarily helpful. Worked within an ongoing therapeutic relationship, one notices that there is a lot that swims under the surface in an EMDR session that's worth examination later in the ordinary work of therapy. The other thing one notices is how when used in an established therapeutic relationship the survivor's impulse toward narrative is strong. Surfacing from a saccade of eye movement or some other form of bilateral stimulation, they are more likely to want one to witness their experience, and to give detailed verbal expression to where they are at in the unfolding scenes. On the other hand, a young man, traumatized by his journey to the West and unable to talk was helped simply because the method allows the survivor to share very little. How does it work? My instinct is to understand it as resetting communication deep in the brain stem, allowing us to venture through the forest hunting game like our forebears, bars of light and color playing across our eyes.

Guidance

Measures of Traumatic Stress

Psychological measures of traumatic stress can be enormously helpful in orienting psychotherapists to bodily reactions and to wider psychological responses to trauma, and are certainly good learning tools that used diligently and critically sink into a general awareness of what one might be alert to in the assessment and ongoing work with a survivor.

Of particular value are:

Clinician Administered PTSD Scale for DSM—5 (CAPS—5) (Weathers et al. 2013).

General Health Questionnaire—28 (GHQ—28) (Goldberg 1978).

Hospital Anxiety and Depression Scale (HADS) (Zigmond and Snaith 1983).

Impact of Events Scale (IES) (Weiss and Marmar 1996).

HADS is a very good measure to work through mutually with a stressed colleague because it is good at picking up the hidden anxiety that we may hide from ourselves and each other.

Body Psychotherapies

Fortunately, as we have begun to see the body was not entirely overlooked in psychotherapy, Wilhelm Reich proposed that psychoanalysis needed to understand how the body creates a defensive muscular armour in response to early trauma. Fritz Perls, the founder of Gestalt Therapy focused on the taste of here and now, and of felt experience, and on the dialogical positioning of the therapist as mentor and guide. This signalled many of the themes that later emerged, as psychotherapy brought the body in from the cold.

Learning Point

Body Oriented Psychotherapies

Pat Ogden—*Sensorimotor Psychotherapy*: uses mindfulness to develop and deepen body awareness of maladaptive responses and work through how we can respond in careful and gradual ways. Her sensorimotor psychotherapy for treating trauma integrates bottom up and top down approaches directly. Broadly speaking, she works on three levels: cognitive, emotional, and sensorimotor which correspond to our three levels of brain architecture neo-mammalian, mammalian and reptilian. So for example, she will notice a client's physical response, and ask what is it telling you? A clenched fist might indicate anger, a dropped head not wanting to be noticed because that would make you too vulnerable. And this can lead to experimenting with different ways of being, or to other memories, which can then become available events for processing.

Peter Levine—*Somatic Experiencing* understands how our emotional-physiological regulatory responses can become stuck and uses an understanding of how prey animals utilize these physical energies to discharge bodily energy and stay in balance. His method using his techniques of titration, working with tiny bits of traumatic experience at a time, and gradually introducing more and pendulation, moving between arousal and calm to help clients work through their somatic trauma.

Stephen Porges—*Polyvagal Theory* understands and works with the sympathetic and parasympathetic nervous system and an awareness of the pathway of the vagal nerve through the body and our physiological interactions with it. Tracks how our bodies and brains interact with one another to regulate our physiological states, and focuses on ways the nervous system can re-regulate. Steven Porges polyvagal theory has greatly contributed to this field of neuroscientific research. He speaks of how on a neural level not just the brain but the entire nervous system is altered by trauma. The dorsal vagal nerve shuts us down, whereas the ventral branch serves the social engagement system (governing facial muscles): that which is playful and wants to engage. He discovered if you activate this system though providing safety you can reach the client much more quickly, so the client-therapist positive relationship is crucial.

What emerges in the work of others such as Pat Ogden, Stephen Porges, Peter Levine, and Janina Fischer are powerfully real and metaphorical ways of engaging with the body, and any serious work with trauma needs to engage with these ideas. The method that unites these similar although uniquely different approaches is the attention to the bodily state of the survivor, and this followed in a moment by moment unfolding of awareness of body and mind, keeping bodily state and mind connected in the therapeutic work, and the warm attentive, intimate disposition of the therapist. Each of these practitioners maintains a professional reserve but this is done with warm engagement. Working with a survivor as he emerged from a long session of work with traumatic memories where we had tracked his powerful somatic responses and his fluctuating capacity to bring his awareness to his experience of massive deregulation, he was amazed at the time that had passed. "You must be so bored witnessing this," he said. "On the contrary," I replied, "I had been watching you just like a parent might have viewed an infant in their cot, with absolutely undivided, and deeply felt, and pleasurable attention."

Mindfulness

Mindfulness has made a powerful contribution to this new paradigm, this has emerged among others from the work of Jon Kabbat-Zinn (1990), providing programs to cope with physical and emotional pain, anxiety, stress, and panic. These are matters that are understood as having shared reality between the inner world and the outer world. Almost subversively, mindfulness makes no distinction between inner and outer, although it pays close attention to the survivors felt experience. A cornerstone of mindfulness practice is the body scan, practiced everyday, this draws our attention to the closely observed sensations that unfold in our body, it teaches us to be tolerant of what we might otherwise describe as pain or discomfort or suffering. It asks us to be curious of what arises, of how our attention narrows when we encounter emotional or physical pain, of how these are closely related, of how we habitually withdraw rather than being curious and paying attention. Through this process, it invites us to understand the subtle grammar of the body-mind. Eventually, we come almost full circle with the psychotherapies in the work of John Welwood and Daniel Seigal and others. John Welwood synthesizes the work of Eugene Gendlin (1996) in focusing and felt experience. This makes use of a closely observed phenomenological method to watch how as emotional experience is attended to in the moment, and allowed to unfold, deeper resonances, meanings and experience emerge, in what can be described as a felt shift. Welwood relates this profound form of attention back to the serendipitous coming together of his psychological studies and the Buddhist path. He writes that this involves directly opening to whatever experience is at hand, rather than stepping back from it, and engaging in a dialogical inquiry, or allowing the unfolding of the felt meanings within it (Welwood 1996) In this approach, one directly recognizes and meets one's experience as it is, without concern for what it means, where it comes from, or where it leads. "There is no reinforcement of an observing self trying to grasp, understand, or come to terms with some observed content of consciousness" (Welwood 1996, p. 108). Embodied in this approach described in the same paper is "finding the right distance from feeling", and this summarizes much of the new embodied work with trauma.

Learning Point

Embodied in this approach is "finding the right distance from feeling" and this summarises much of the new embodied work with trauma.

By contrast, Daniel Seigal swims in the same sea influenced by colleagues such as Jon Kabat-Zinn and Jack Kornfield who sit within the Southern Buddhist schools and he brings to our attention the delightful manner in which the ancient philosophical traditions and practices of mindfulness that have recently sprung up in the West coincide with the emerging field of Western neuropsychology and neurophysiology. His approach can be summarized by the notion of "mindsight." This takes a view of mind that experiences itself both as located within but also simultaneously existing way beyond a confined sense of self. This entails being able to swim in and out of an expansive field of consciousness, participating freely in big mind and little mind (Siegel 2011). In such a state of mind, he invites us to become our own best friends, such an approach invites compassion toward self, which opens a fertile process of discovery for the traumatized.

Family Therapy

How does all this coincide with systemic family therapy? We can turn to Gregory Bateson and the notion that supremely for him, mind was immanent in all things and that our downfall is to constantly work as if we are either at the center or even more dangerously in control of the cybernetics of reality, whereas it is all deeply complex. The wisest course is to take as reflexive a stance as possible, although this too is necessarily impossible because the web of systems of which we are a part is infinite. Out of this emerges what Barry Mason (1993) describes as the notion of safe uncertainty, in the face of never being able to encompass the whole of a situation, how to describe the limits within which we can safely negotiate reality. Humility and openness to other people's ideas lived experience is necessarily part of this process. There is a danger of throwing the baby out with the bathwater and moving into a philosophical position wherein all knowledge and expertise is given up as partial and the best we can manage is to perturb the systems in which we live, and breathe and work. What is noticeable at this moment is how absent the body is from systemic family therapy, the debate is fixated on how we position ourselves within an epistemological system, and this is a long way from trauma. Against this, we can propose a semi-realist position, akin in many respects to the Madhyamaka school of Buddhist philosophy. This proposes that all phenomena are empty of inherent existence, but in that very emptiness, they are substantially pregnant with possibility. This being so every possible aspect of experience contains both a substantial presence, and at the very same time, the seeds of its extinction out of which flow infinite possibilities.

Family Therapy has had its body practitioners, the early Structural Family Therapists, such as Salvador Minuchin were keenly aware of the body as a presence in the work. However, the vigor and delicacy with which Minuchin wrestled with the manifestations of family structures and bodily presentations such as anorexia, and the paradoxes of highly controlling enfeeblement were often experienced as controversial and out of step with therapy's shift toward second-order thinking. Always some-what allergic to affect, and with the body already only faintly present, it almost evaporated in the debate about meaning that ensued. Is it, that in order to grow up conceptually, particularly in Britain and America, that intellectual knowledge, and conceptual finesse have to be demonstrated as having primacy rather than the body?

It is feminist practitioners who most elegantly brought intellect, conceptual finesse, and the body together. Consider for example Gillian Walker and Virginia Goldner writing about the wounded prince and the women who love him (1995). Here there is attention to the body, and to powerful feelings. There is also as the work opens the paradoxical absence of the feminine body as a power to itself. The work of therapy is an encouragement of the emergence of autonomy and partnership, in which themes of intimacy and attachment are deeply explored, and the cultural frame, always likely to entrap women, is critiqued and subverted to therapeutic advantage. The work of Yvonne Dolan (1991) should also form a centerpiece to systemic work with trauma. Even before our deep-ened understanding of neuroscience and bodily processes, she attended to work with adult survivors of sexual abuse with delicacy and strength, deeply understanding the fluctuating capacity of the survivor to stay with the transformation of experience that imperils us. The other outstanding systemic work with survivors is that of Inger Agger, described in *The Blue Room* (1994). Here she creates a house for women where each room has a symbolic meaning connected with experience and the body. As work progresses the house and each room takes on the metaphor of the body itself, as container and witness of experience.

What seems true here is that as attachment has landed among systemic family therapy, there have been some fascinating departures from the meaning-centered approach to systemic work. Take for instance the ways that Rudi Dallos and Arlene Vetere have mapped out a compelling vision of intervention in *Systemic Therapy and Attachment Narratives* (2009). What they have joined up is the feeling space, the limbic system, our ways of attaching and detaching, and how disjointed narratives of family life are faced, worked through, and made more coherent within the containment of a systemic scaffolding.

All of this work would seem almost in vain if we did not recognize the social contexts of work, as so much systemic therapy does. Here we can think of the gentle, tough, collaborative work of Lynne Hoffman in *Exchanging Voices* (1993) taking the position of elder in work across generations in a community. What also leaps to mind is the deeply passionate work of Just Therapy weaving together themes of social justice and family therapy in their work in Lower Hutt, New Zealand (White 1990).

Finally, there is a debt to the practitioners of psychoanalytic family therapy who are alive to the inner turn. To Sally Box and colleagues demonstrating the therapist at work in their body in the here and now of family sessions, a description which falls far short of the elegant complexity they bring to the work. Also to John Schlapobersky and Robyn Skynner (1987b), who kept the link between the systemic and the psychoanalytic alive with their pithy attention to the emotional life of families in therapy. In addition, there is John Schlapobersky's penetrating work with groups and the group analytic and systemic understanding of how group dynamics run through families, and family dynamics resonate through groups. Informing this, there is a deep appreciation of the capacity of groups to engage deeply with profound emotional experience and of the group as container and witness and transformer of bodily experience (2016).

Integration in Theory and Practice

What all the above invites is the question as to how the insights from these different paradigms can be integrated. In what follows there is the suggestion of a way forward if we start with the ideas that each of these different approaches to psychotherapy suggests about integration as a psychological process. In the Western tradition there is an assumption that healthy development tends strongly toward integration. For instance, within the Kleinian tradition there is the notion that the paranoid-schizoid and depressive positions are in a continual flux of integration and disintegration, but that they tend toward resolution and integration throughout life; within the Jungian tradition there is the belief that individuation is a process whereby the shadow and denied aspects of self are integrated so that the individuated self comes to contain the whole of a life; within the Person-Centred tradition there is the idea that the harmonious self emerges from the non-defensive integration of visceral, sensory, and emotional experience; within the Systemic tradition there is the idea that resolution emerges from a circular process whereby multiple views of self are integrated; within Mindfulness there is the sense that, emptied of obstructive anxieties, we can be offered the serene experience of allowing all experience to register as self. However, although psychological integration is a goal in each of these ways of working they tend to remain self-referential, and largely enclosed within their own systems of thought. Furthermore, and most importantly, because no one paradigm can adequately deliver everyone from trauma, we need a supra-paradigmatic working definition of integration that can speak across the boundaries of different psychological approaches. Most importantly, because trauma is a disintegrative experience, integration and reintegration need to be conceived not merely as psychological processes but ones that incorporates multiple levels of context. As each of the foregoing chapters has attempted to show psychological experiences are embedded within social, cultural, and political systems that shape, constrain, and amplify personal experience.

What follows is an attempt to formulate a model of thinking that can integrate different psychological paradigms. The fundamental idea emerges from the notion of Holons, which Arthur Koestler invented, and which Ken Wilbur the American philosopher has elaborated probably to its fullest extent (Wilbur 2000) within the larger framework of his lifetimes work on Integral Theory. According to Wilbur a holon is both a thing in itself and simultaneously carries within itself a pattern, or imprint or code of the larger whole of which it is part. A family relationship understood to be isomorphic is a systemic version of this idea. The interesting thing about holons and isomorphic patterns is that they exist in reality, but also as principles, philosophical abstractions, and guiding metaphors. They have a protean quality that carry within themselves the seeds of what will emerge as a pattern of what went before. If we hold this quality in mind and turn to the different concepts of integration offered above from the differing psychological models and conceive of them not only as discrete ideas of integration but also as holons of an integrative conception of human development something interesting begins to emerge that can speak powerfully to the disintegrative effects of trauma. The diagram below might serve to illustrate its potential (Fig. 12.1).

In the diagram the outer circle represents disintegration, the inner circle represents integration and a more inclusive, holarchic vision. The four quadrants group together aspects of psychological models, themes from attachment theory, social-cultural experience and trauma. The values denoted in the outer perimeter of the circle are negative and disintegrative, and each of these negative disintegrative values has a corresponding positive and integrative and value as one moves into the center

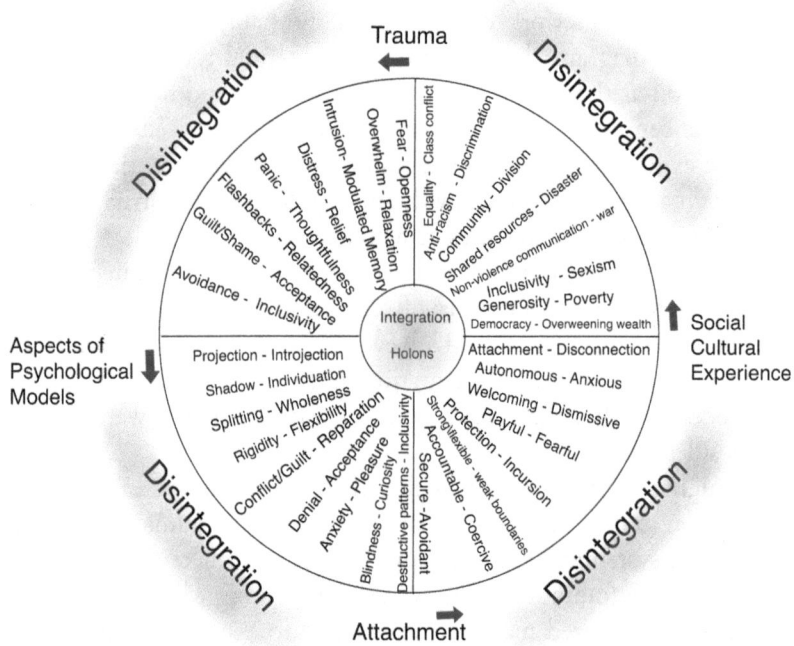

Fig. 12.1 Disintegration-integration holarchy

of the circle toward an inclusive and holarchic vision. Values in the outer circle have an equivalence insofar as they are divisive, and troubling. In contrast, values at the center are unifying.

What the model suggest is that the negative terms in the outer ring can be read across the quadrant they reside in as having an equivalence to disintegrative values in another quadrant. For instance, if we take a psychological term such as projection it can be understood across the divide in the social and cultural experience quadrant as having an equivalence to division or even warfare, insofar as war promotes strong "us and them" experiences. Or we can take a term like inflexibility and relate it across to overweening wealth in the opposite quadrant, insofar as huge wealth tends to create social systems that are protective of the privileges of creating wealth and militate against the flexibility that enable social systems to evolve toward greater equality. We can also see how the concepts and experiences in the quadrant of trauma like fear, relate across the divide to the opposite quadrant, where to be coercive within an attachment framework emerges from the habitual need to manage hostility. The diagram also illustrates the potential for movement from disintegration at the periphery toward integration and holarchic experience at the center. Furthermore, in the impulse toward integration and holarchic experience there is a self-fulfilling unifying potential insofar as things such as introjection, individuation, pleasure, inclusivity, curiosity, and plasticity are characteristics of wholeness.

One of the dangers of this approach is of falling into category error where a concept from one order of reasoning is treated unambiguously as being equivalent to another. However, if the movements from disintegration and trauma toward integration and wholeness are characterized as a processes rather than fixed concepts the tendency toward category error is sidestepped.

We might wonder how this highly theoretical take on integration of theories play out in the practice of working with trauma. An example from within systemic family therapy practice will make this clearer. For instance, a team found itself deeply divided working with a family where the deeply traumatized male partner seemed to experience such massive terror that he just couldn't allow his partner and children to leave his side. He was, from one perspective, dominating his family with gendered oppression, from another he was like a helpless child who had trapped his family in a life cycle transition, preventing any of them from moving on and leaving home. These were not mutually exclusive hypotheses but the strength of feeling caused disorder in the team who were usually excellent at cultivating curiosity and allowing for difference. A visiting colleague wondered if the team conflict that had broken out had taken on the characteristic of an oedipal clash where powerful emotions were being evoked by the man that prevented what was in the mind of one set of colleagues being gathered up in minds of the other set of colleagues. This intervention revived the team's curiosity and together they wondered if the man's limbic experience of terror was so acute that he was literally unable to think, and this unthinking quality had infiltrated team dynamics. At this moment we can see that each of these descriptions fall within the traumatic unintegrated periphery of the holistic and integrative perspective on trauma in the diagram above. However, just being able to hold an experience as a process rather than a thing in itself, or a position to be defended at all costs, allows it to shift toward an integrated and holarchic perspective. From that holarchic center all positions seem more deeply contingent, they do not lose definition but nevertheless they take on a perspective of fluidity, they become provisional, and negotiable, rigorous in what they have to offer but no longer hard and fast truths.

Here is an example from the holarchic center—psychoanalytic colleagues were persuaded by other practitioners to take their practice out of the clinic and into schools where the psychosocial aspects of trauma were vividly available to be worked with, and where practitioners from other disciplines were readily accepted into the team, and their perspectives in supervision and consultation were welcomed. What this final example demonstrates is that in the movement in healing from trauma from the disintegrated periphery to the holarchic center there is a transcendent edge that many survivors recognize, that we are not alone with our experience, and it is the perspectives that embody multitudes of experience that come closest to capturing the journey into, and out the other side of trauma.

In my practice a deeply holarchic moment was years ago while reading Mary Main (1991) on attachment. I was thunderstruck by the parallel that emerged between the way very young children are unable to be metacognitive and the clinical experience of working with incredibly sophisticated survivors of trauma who were equally unable to be metacognitive. This holarchic moment created an arc that enabled me to relate themes in attachment theory, with themes in systemic practice with themes in psychoanalytic practice. The ideas no longer jostled for preeminence, they just settled alongside each other in the pleasure of holarchic vision.

What we learn from the holarchic center is that the tight boundaries of intellectual disciplines can be given up in a virtuous manner so that our psychological work is informed by many different ways of thinking. For instance, an insight from mindfulness inspired CBT that we are not our thoughts and our mind like a fridge is not all the things it contains can be the concrete expression that begins to free a person from the terror of their own thinking (Turnbull 2013). The point about the holarchic is that it allows one to relax into ideas and methods that converge and connect. In family therapy the holarchic flavour is deeply conveyed in Giannifranco Cecchin's notion of neutrality being a state curiosity in the observer (Cecchin 1987), where all voices, and especially where all feelings and sensations, are allowed to register in us with bare attention. If this is enlarged to include all theories that coincide and flow through us as we work, registered as hypotheses, and held with an open hand, and understood as process, then we truly arrive at an holoarchic vision. At best the holarchic is transformational: in work with trauma it is an understanding that inhabits many survivors and infiltrates those who work with them, that interconnection is actually a given, and that it has always been there to be seen if we but had the vision to notice it. Once the confining grip of bodily limbic terror has been loosened reflection allows us to see that the experience of trauma that robbed us of connection, in shocking and unexpected ways, allows us to appreciate and deeply savor interconnectedness in ways that can be transformational.

Finale

What this book has set out to encourage is for survivors, their family's friends, for therapists and practitioners to take the inner turn. Hopefully what we have seen is that the inner turn is not an abstract place, it is somewhere deep within us, an embodied feeling place. Furthermore, there are things of the heart, that peculiar place of trauma that resonate simultaneously with the sense of extinction and infinite possibility. Working through a shattering trauma that was barely acknowledged at the time, a survivor described being tasked to recover his comrades' bodies from a crash site. This set him off on a life course, which in later years revisited with panic attacks and terror of death. After a session of therapeutic work, he said to me, "After that session I had a sense of being in that aeroplane in which my friends had died, coming into land as they had been. Looking out of the window as it tilted toward the airport where their families were waiting for them was undoubtedly a peak experience. Then forty five seconds of terror as the plane plunged out of control and into the woods. But on this occasion I was not terrified as usual when these memories and sensations returned but just delightfully there, in ways I cannot explain but that feel deeply transformative."

These are not rare insights, in some way, they are simultaneously both the ordinary and extraordinary consequences of trauma: we are put in touch with our extinction, and through work that can allow us finally to re-experience our body not as a source of terror, but as a source of curiosity, wounded though it may be, we find ourselves immersed in the fabric not only of own lives but the substance of everyone else's. Able to see the fear and terror from which we readily withdraw with wide-open eyes; also able to experience simple joys, perhaps even the sense that things are lit from within; this is where work with families is invited: knowing that it is possible to slow down the pace of a session, to take the inner turn, to settle into just this moment and pursue detail by detail the felt experience of a family member, and then how it resonates around the family in a circular fashion, who most identifies, who is repelled into flight or pulled back by curiosity, what is shared and what is singularly one person's experience, what joins them and what separates? The wonder of reflexivity and circularity is that they can encompass all of this, and more.

References

Agger, Inger. 1994. *The Blue Room: Trauma and Testimony Among Refugee Women*. London: Zed Press.

Bick, Esther. 1988. The Experience of Skin in Early Object Relations. In *Melanie Klein Today: Volume 1, Mainly Theory*, ed. Elizabeth Bott-Spillius. London: Brunner Routledge.

Blackwell, Dick. 1997. Holding, Containing and Bearing Witness: The Problem of Helpfulness in Encounters with Torture Survivors. *Journal of Social Work Practice* 11 (2): 81–89.

Bléandonu, Gérard. 1994. *Wilfrid Bion: His Life and Work 1897–1979*. London: Free Association Books.

Caruth, Cathy (ed.). 1995. *Trauma: Explorations in Memory*. Baltimore: John Hopkins University Press.

Cecchin, Gianfranco. 1987. Hypothesizing, Circularity, and Neutrality Revisited: An Invitation to Curiosity. *Family Process* 26: 405–413.

Dolan, Yvonne. 1991. *Resolving Sexual Abuse: Solution-Focused Therapy and Ericksonian Hypnosis for Adult Survivors*. New York: Norton.

Fonagy, Peter, György Gergely, Elliot Juris, and Mary Target. 2002. *Affect Regulation, Mentalization, and the Development of the Self*. New York: Other Press.

Gay, Peter. 1988. *Freud: A Life for Our Time*. New York: Norton.

Gendlin, Eugene. 1996. *Focusing-Oriented Psychotherapy: A Manual of the Experiential Method*. London: Guilford Press.

Goldberg, D. 1978. *Manual of the General Health Questionnaire*. Windsor: NFER-Nelson.

Hoffman, Lyn. 1993. *Exchanging Voices*. London: Karnac.

Jones, Ernest. 1961. *The Life and Work of Sigmund Freud*. London: Hogarth Press.

Kabat-Zinn, Jon. 1990. *Full Catastrophe Living: How to Cope with Stress, Pain and Illness Using Mindfulness Meditation*. London: Piatkus.

Kurzweil, Edith. 1989. *The Freudians*. New Haven: Yale University Press.

Laub, Dori. 1995. Truth and Testimony: The Process and the Struggle. In *Trauma: Explorations in Memory*, ed. Cathy Caruth. Baltimore: John Hopkins University Press.

Laub, Dori, and Nanette Auerhahn. 1993. Knowing and Not Knowing Massive Psychic Trauma: Forms of Traumatic Memory. *International Journal of Psychoanalysis* 74: 287–302.

Levy, Susan. 2004. Containment and Validation: Working with Survivors of Trauma. In *The Perversion of Loss: Psychoanalytic Perspectives on Trauma*, ed. Susan Levy and Alexandra Lemma. London: Whurr.

Main, Mary. 1991. Metacognitive Knowledge, Metacognitive Monitoring, and Singular (Coherent) vs. Multiple (Incoherent) Model of Attachment: Findings and Directions for Future Research. In *Attachment Across the Life Cycle*, ed. Colin Murray-Parkes, Joan Stevenson-Hinde, and Peter Harris. London: Routledge.

Mason, Barry. 1993. Towards Positions of Safe Uncertainty. *Human Systems* 4: 189–200.

Pines, Dinora. 1994. *A Woman's Unconscious Use of Her Body*. New Haven: Yale University Press.

Rothschild, Babette. 2010. *8 Keys to Safe Trauma Recovery*. London: Norton.

Schlapobersky, John. 2016. *From the Couch to the Circle*. London: Routledge.

Shephard, Ben. 2000. *A War of Nerves*. London: Jonathan Cape.

Skynner, Robin. 1987a. *Explorations with Families: Group Analysis and Family Therapy*. London: Routledge.

Skynner, Robyn. 1987b. An Open-Systems Group-Analytic Approach to Family Therapy. In Robyn Skynner, *Explorations with Families: Group Analysis and Family Therapy*, ed. John Schlapobersky. London: Routledge.

Siegel, Daniel. 2011. *Mindsight: Transform Your Brain with the New Science of Kindness*. London: Oneworld.

Stanton, Martin. 2002. The Love/Hate Couple in the Primal Scene: The Problem of Dyads and Triads in Relationship Therapy. In *Love and Hate: Psychoanalytic Perspectives*, ed. David Mann. London: Brunner-Routledge.

Turnbull, Dheeresh. 2013. *The CBT-Pot: Learning to Play Your Mind*. Brighton: Pen Press.

Van der Kolk, Bessel. 1987. *Psychological Trauma*. Washington: American Psychological Press.

Van der Kolk, Bessel. 2015. *The Body Keeps the Score*. London: Penguin.

Walker, Gillian, and Virginia Goldner. 1995. The Wounded Prince and the Women Who Love Him. In *Gender, Power and Relationships*, ed. Charlotte Burck and Bebe Speed. London: Routledge.

Weathers, F.W., D.D. Blake, P.P. Schnurr, D.G. Kaloupek, B.P. Marxand, and T.M. Keane. 2013. *The Clinician-Administered PTSD Scale for DSM-5 (CAPS-5)*. https://www.ptsd.va.gov/professional/assessment/adult-int/cap s.asp.

Weiss, D.S., and C.R. Marmar. 1996. The Impact of Event Scale—Revised. In *Assessing Psychological Trauma and PTSD*, ed. J. Wilson and T.M. Keane, 399–411. New York: Guilford.

Welwood, John. 1996. Reflection and Presence: The Dialectic of Self Knowledge. *The Journal of Transpersonal Psychology* 28: 107–128.

White, Cheryl (ed.). 1990. *Social Justice and Family Therapy* (Dulwich Centre Newsletter, No. 1).

Wilbur, Ken. 2000. *A Brief History of Everything*. Dublin: Gateway.

Woodcock, Jeremy. 1997. Groupwork with Refugees and Asylum Seekers. In *Race and Groupwork*, ed. Allan Brown and Tara Mistry. London: Whiting and Birch.

Woodcock, Jeremy. 2001. Being, Noticing, Knowing: The Emergence of Resilience in Groupwork. In *Strengthening Resiliency Through Group Work*, ed. Tim Kelly, Toby Berman-Rossi, and Susanne Palombo. New York: Haworth Press.

Zigmond, A.S., and R.P. Snaith. 1983. The Hospital Anxiety and Depression Scale. *Acta Psychiatrica Scand* 67: 361–370.

Zulueta, Felicity de. 1993. *From Pain to Violence: The Traumatic Roots of Destructiveness*. London: Whurr.

Zulueta, Felicity de. 2004. Human Violence is a Preventable Disease. In *Attachment and Human Survival*, ed. Marci Green and Marc Scholes. London: Karnac.

Index

© The Editor(s) (if applicable) and The Author(s), under exclusive license to Springer Nature Switzerland AG 2022
J. Woodcock, *Families and Individuals Living with Trauma*,
Palgrave Texts in Counselling and Psychotherapy,
https://doi.org/10.1007/978-3-030-79039-4